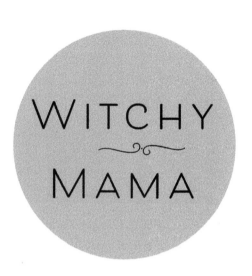

WITCHY

MAMA

About the Authors

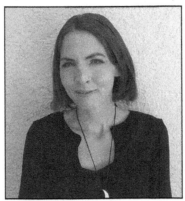

Melanie Marquis is the creator of the *Modern Spellcaster's Tarot* (illustrated by Scott Murphy) and the author of several books, including *A Witch's World of Magick*, *The Witch's Bag of Tricks*, *Beltane*, and *Lughnasadh*. The founder of United Witches Global Coven and a local coordinator for the Pagan Pride Project, she loves sharing magick with others and has presented workshops and rituals to audiences across the US. She lives in Denver, Colorado, and can be found online at MelanieMarquis.com.

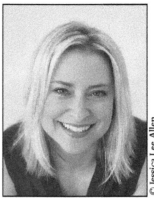

Emily A. Francis is a clinical massage therapist who holds a bachelor's degree in exercise science and wellness. She is also a certified pediatric massage therapist and the author of *Stretch Therapy* (Blue River Press, 2012) and an upcoming book on the emotional muscle body to be published by Llewellyn in 2017. Her writing has been featured in publications including *TODAY Parents, Fit Pregnancy,* and *Massage Magazine.* She lives in Atlanta, Georgia, and can be found online at EmilyAFrancisBooks.com.

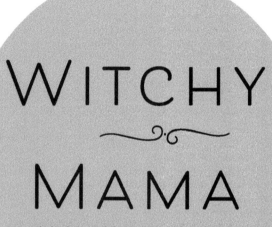

WITCHY

MAMA

Magickal Traditions, Motherly Insights
& Sacred Knowledge

MELANIE MARQUIS
EMILY A. FRANCIS

Llewellyn Publications
Woodbury, Minnesota

First Edition
Third Printing, 2018

Cover art: iStockphoto.com/63005403©sergeytitov1977
iStockphoto.com/32196582©Richard Ellgen
iStockphoto.com/32198172©Richard Ellgen
iStockphoto.com/6107557©mugshot
Cover design: Ellen Lawson
Interior Photographs © Jessica Lee Allen

Llewellyn is a registered trademark of Llewellyn Worldwide Ltd.

Library of Congress Cataloging-in-Publication Data
Names: Marquis, Melanie, 1976– author.
Title: Witchy mama : magickal traditions, motherly insights & sacred
  knowledge / by Melanie Marquis and Emily A. Francis.
Description: First Edition. | Woodbury, MN : Llewellyn Publications, 2016. |
  Includes bibliographical references and index.
Identifiers: LCCN 2016002266 (print) | LCCN 2016009924 (ebook) | ISBN
  9780738748306 | ISBN 9780738749105 ()
Subjects: LCSH: Pregnancy—Popular works. | Childbirth—Popular works. |
  Magic.
Classification: LCC RG551 .M37 2016 (print) | LCC RG551 (ebook) | DDC
  618.2—dc23
LC record available at http://lccn.loc.gov/2016002266

Llewellyn Publications
A Division of Llewellyn Worldwide Ltd.
2143 Wooddale Drive
Woodbury, MN 55125-2989
www.llewellyn.com

Printed in the United States of America

Other Books by Melanie Marquis

Beltane

Lughnasadh

A Witch's World of Magick

The Witch's Bag of Tricks

Modern Spellcaster's Tarot

Carl Llewellyn Weschcke

Other Books by Emily A. Francis

Stretch Therapy
(Blue River Press, 2012)

Dedication

This book is lovingly dedicated to our sacred children, who are our greatest treasures, and to all the good mamas of the past, present, and future, including our own.

Acknowledgments

Special thanks to Jessica Allen, Colette Shorthouse, Stephanie Colletti, Johns Creek Yoga Studio, Roz Zollinger, Claire Marie Miller, Jill Kostrinsky, and Jorja Fleming for your help and contributions. We would also like to thank everyone at Llewellyn who helped make this book possible. Emily would like to give special thanks to the girls who made her a mother, Hannah and Ava, and infinite gratitude to her whole incredible family for all their love, kindness, and support. Melanie would like to give thanks to her children, Aidan and Mia, who make her laugh and smile every single day.

Contents

Being open to the many options and possibilities available to you will help increase your chances of bringing into your life the child of your dreams. Discover tips for opening your mind, body, and spirit to conception, explore fertility charms and symbols from around the world, create your very own fertility altar, and more.

From setting boundaries to setting intentions, this chapter will help you face fears and overcome other challenges to help you embrace and enjoy your pregnancy, swollen ankles and all.

Discover easy-to-learn stretches, yoga poses, visualizations, and other activities that can greatly reduce the physical discomfort of pregnancy.

Every mama is different, and you will be a mama like no other. This chapter will help you embrace and empower your maternal instincts to help you be the best mom you can be, right from the start. Explore the mother archetype in many varied forms, try exercises and visualizations to awaken your inner strength and confidence, and discover ways to communicate and bond with your baby pre-birth.

Chapter 5: **Pregnancy Dreams Deciphered** 67

Ask any pregnant woman and she'll tell you that you're not alone in having those super-bizarre, wild, and vivid dreams. From dreaming you've given birth to another species to dreaming you're literally as fat as a house, learn how to interpret those often mixed-up, messed-up pregnancy dreams.

Chapter 6: **Preparing for Birth** 83

Learn how to make childbearing a little more bearable with simple visualizations, meditations, breathing techniques, charms, rituals, and other strategies for easing the pains of giving birth and for promoting a safe and speedy delivery.

Chapter 7: **Welcoming Baby** 99

Discover traditional birth rituals for blessing your baby and explore time-honored charms for soothing colic, gathered from folk magick traditions around the world. Learn easy-to-use pediatric massage moves to help relieve baby's gas, and glean some straightforward, practical advice on nursing.

Chapter 8: **Baby Astrology** 117

Read about your baby's zodiac sign and discover their lucky colors, lucky animals, and more.

Chapter 9: **Relaxation Tools for Moms** 131

Learn breathing exercises for calming the mind, discover the top ten stones and scents to soothe your nerves, explore calming meditations and visualizations you can use for in-the-moment stress relief or as an everyday way to maintain your calm, and relax in the peace and solitude of a ritual bath.

Chapter 10: **Energizing Techniques for Moms** 149

Master easy movements for energizing the mind and body, discover energizing herbal scents, stones, and colors, explore a sampling of meditations and visualizations designed to increase your energy, and more.

From scents and sounds to colors and crystals, discover ways to make your little one's bath time more magickal.

Learn how to use massage and touch to encourage baby to relax, and discover magickal charms, scents, and colors that help promote good dreams and a restful night's sleep.

Master special techniques for bringing out the magick in food while you slice, stir, or mash, and learn how to make your own food for baby.

Learn how to make the nursery, your own bedroom, and all the rest of your home a place of magick. From practical tips and charms for combating clutter and fending off negative vibes to techniques using plants, scents, crystals, and feng shui, you'll discover lots of ways to infuse your home with positive energy and keep it safe and welcoming for all who dwell there.

Discover ways to strengthen your psychic abilities and hone your mother's intuition, and explore a sampling of divination tools useful for moms at any stage along the journey.

For many moms, personal appearance isn't exactly at the top of the priority list, but just because you're covered in baby slobber doesn't mean you can't look and feel your best, every day. In this chapter, you'll discover some beauty secrets to help you be just as beautiful on the outside as you are on the inside.

Learn new ways to fuel your passions, explore simple techniques of sex magick, discover the top ten stones for promoting love and romance, and more.

Discover fun ways to nurture your child's psychic development, learn how to make some cool, kid-friendly magickal crafts, and master simple charms to help ease the pain of boo-boos and other mild kid disasters.

Learn how to keep your dreams alive and increase your chances of achieving them, and discover some simple tips for fitting physical exercise and self-care into your busy life as a mom.

Figures

Foreword by Emily

The first time I got pregnant, I was excited but a little uncertain. I wasn't ready to look at my pregnancy as some wonderful, magickal experience... yet. But after suffering a miscarriage late in the first trimester, my attitude changed completely. I went from feeling ambivalent about even being pregnant to feeling terrified, wanting it, not wanting it, questioning it, loving it, not believing entirely that it was really real, being excited, and then feeling loss and pain. The loss shook me to my very core. I woke up every night after finding out we lost it and would roll over and lie on my husband and just cry. Oh, what I would have given to have never doubted, never questioned, never been negative! Oh, what I would have done to have another chance to get pregnant and have a baby! I would do it all right this time!

Shortly after suffering that loss, I was in my yoga class, lying in *savasana*, the relaxation pose. As I lay there, still and quiet, I heard a voice as clear as day whisper in my ear, "Are you ready now? Because there is a little girl trying to come through." I answered with all my heart and soul to that voice: "Yes, yes, yes, I am *ready*!" I went home and told my husband, "We are having a girl!" He asked me, "Are we pregnant?" and I said, "Not yet." But soon we were.

And thus began my own journey. Not to spoil the ending, but I loved it all. Every step of the way, I loved it all. Those harder days when I was so sick to my stomach that I had to be dragged into a medical center to get fluids? Even those I loved. And oh my universe, that day they laid that baby girl on my chest? No one in the world has ever managed to adequately describe that moment when you see your newborn baby for the very first time. It's because it is simply not possible. You just have to experience it yourself.

As I write this today, I am the mother of a wonderful twenty-month-old girl and one week away from delivering my second miracle. As I sit here heavily pregnant and in my most vulnerable place, I figure this is the best time to be as honest as I can with you. Conception has its many challenges, pregnancy does too but in a totally different way, and motherhood … well, that is a prize beyond comprehension until you get there. There are no words that do it justice, so I won't try.

When you are expecting, everyone will offer you a book—maybe even this one. But in regard to this book and every other book out there about pregnancy, conception, and motherhood, I offer you this as the most sincere and loving advice that I can possibly offer: *Trust your own instincts above all else.*

Don't let what we say in this book, as well as what anyone says in any book or article, beat out the voice in your own head and gut.

Motherhood is amazing, without a doubt. Being pregnant is phenomenal, but it's also a challenge. It's not all rainbows and butterflies. It hurts. Your body goes through a huge transformation—but it's for the greatest reason known to humankind!

One of our primary purposes in writing this book is to help you realize the incredible journey you are on while you are still on it. Many people look back with great regret for not embracing the moments when they were actually *in* each of these moments. I'm in my late thirties, and I think with that comes a very different perspective about pregnancy. As I've shared my complete joy and appreciation for this gift of pregnancy and motherhood, I've received a lot of letters from women saying they wish they would have been more like me during the times they carried their children. They look back and realize how much of it was spent complaining and trying to hurry up time. Now they wish with everything in them that time would slow down. I want to bring you into the present moment of exactly where you are. Whether you currently are pregnant, are a mom, are at the very beginning of this journey, or are contemplating trying to get pregnant, I want you to be here for it. Each stage has great offerings. I want to help you be open to them all.

So come along with me. The best is yet to be.

Love,

Emily

Foreword by Melanie

I've never considered myself to be the domestic type. While I might like to watch Donna Reed or Martha Stewart on television, I don't exactly measure up to these standards. When I found out I was pregnant with my first child, I completely flipped out, instantly knowing that this was something I simply could not do. I was no mother! I was still just trying to grow up, having recently left my partying years behind. I knew absolutely nothing about babies, I was terrible at housekeeping, and I basically only ever cooked Ramen noodles or macaroni and cheese. I just couldn't see myself succeeding in the role of the traditional mother.

I was on birth control pills when I got pregnant. In fact, I found out about the pregnancy when I went to the doctor to get my prescription refilled. I hadn't missed any pills, but I had been a few hours late in taking them a couple of times. I didn't think it was that big of a deal, until the doctor came in and told me she couldn't give me any more birth control pills because I was already pregnant!

I was in total shock. So much so that I was too embarrassed and frightened to tell anyone, even the father, who was my steady boyfriend (and now husband) at the time. I kept the secret to myself as long as I could, spending hours each day trying to figure out how I could break the news and reminding myself that I couldn't keep putting it off. I knew I was being stupid, but I just couldn't bring myself to say anything.

When I finally did tell the father, he was surprised, but happy and accepting. I think it was something he had always wanted but maybe didn't want to admit. Once my news was out, I found that the pressure and anxiety instantly lifted, and I began to open myself to that motherly love that had been building up and brewing within me.

My nesting instincts kicked in, and I found myself blessed with this incredible power to get things organized, prepared, and taken care of like never before (and never since!). By the time I was pretty far along in my pregnancy, I felt like I was fairly prepared. It still wasn't something I was totally excited about, but I had accepted my fate and I was determined to make the most of it.

And then he arrived. My precious Aidan, my son. Words do no justice to that moment when you look into those shining eyes of your child for the very first time. All the fears and doubts I had were instantly blown away. At that moment, I knew that I wanted and would do no less than protect this boy and nurture this boy and love this boy every single day that I'm on this earth. In that moment, I embraced my mommy-self to the fullest.

Six years later, my daughter Mia was born. She, too, was a surprise! Having had the failure with birth control pills, I had switched to another birth control method that was given through a shot once every several months. I was six days late getting my shot, and those six short days were apparently too long to wait. I was pregnant, again. And while I was digging being a mom and loving my son, I couldn't imagine going through all those baby and toddler years again. He was just starting to get to the age where he didn't need constant attention, and I had been looking forward to getting a little break. Besides, at that point we knew our son was deaf—he had been born profoundly deaf in both ears—and we had already decided to move across the country so he could have better schooling options than were offered in our area. But now another baby! We were still determined to make the move, and we did. I was eight months pregnant at the time.

That second pregnancy went by in a whirlwind. I had a lot of stress in my life, what with moving across the country, leaving behind friends and family, and also working through some problems in my marriage. I was so stressed about other stuff that I really didn't have time to think too much about the fact that I was pregnant, or to remember to ask myself what in the world was I going to do. Which was probably for the best, because if I had thought about it, I likely would have been even *more* stressed. Before I knew it, I found myself going into labor.

My daughter arrived right on time, beautiful and smiley. I loved her instantly, and I also knew instantly how wrong I had been to doubt that I wanted a second child. I can't imagine not having her, just as I can't imagine not having my son. Though the days get long and the nights even longer sometimes, and though I'm *still* pretty terrible in the domestic duties department, I love being a mom. And I'm a good mom. It's what I am. I just didn't know it.

And I'd be willing to bet that you will be a good mom, too. My hope is that this book will help you enjoy it all to the fullest.

Love,

Melanie

Introduction

Magickal Tools for Making the Most of Motherhood

The journey to parenthood is unique to each individual. For many moms, parenthood is seen as a great blessing, something we've dreamed about, hoped for, and maybe even planned for. For some of us, becoming a parent is a long and challenging road that we achieve only after undergoing fertility treatments or going through the adoption process. For others, the sudden revelation that a new little human is on the way can be surprising, confusing, overwhelming, and maybe even devastating, as our own lives immediately take a back seat to the duties, expectations, and pressures of parenthood.

Whether becoming a parent was an accident or something you went to great lengths to accomplish, you're here now, or you're at least on your way there, so congratulations! As every experienced parent will tell you, you've got a rocky road ahead of you, but it's a delightful journey, nonetheless. While there's no single secret to being a good parent, no specific magick spell to make everything perfect and easy, there are many things you can do to make the most of your experience. We've written this book not to offer parenting advice (you'll get plenty of that as it is) but rather to share with you some effective tools you can use to help your own everyday life as a parent run a little more smoothly and enjoyably. With real talk from real moms coupled with practical tips and techniques for bringing a little more magick into your life, you'll learn how to relieve stress, overcome frustration, increase your energy, relax your body and mind, feed your own passions, and much more.

The book begins with an exploration of your personal journey to parenthood, offering strategies for preparing your body, mind, and spirit for conception, as well as how to care for yourself, set your intentions, and set your boundaries during the early stages of pregnancy. We offer tips for connecting spiritually to your baby pre-birth, simple stretching exercises you can do to help relieve discomfort, and a sampling of magickal tools, rituals, and meditations you can use right now to ease fears, get motivated, and support a successful pregnancy. You'll also find an interpretation guide to those vivid and bizarre dreams that often come with pregnancy. Later in the book you'll find practical, magickal ideas to utilize after your baby arrives and begins growing into a child, from bedtime magick to magickal mealtimes, bathtime magick, playtime magick, relaxing and energizing techniques to keep you feeling your best, tips and tricks for keeping your romantic life alive, magickal beauty tips, psychic development games, strategies for achieving your own dreams, and more.

Feel free to jump around to the sections you need the most right now, or read straight through from the start. We've designed this book to be used as a support and reference you can turn to again and again whenever you need an extra boost of magick to help you along the wild road of life as a parent.

This book will help you to be healthy, mindful, and present to the process of motherhood while encouraging you to grow as an individual. Just as your child grows, so too may your mind and spirit flourish and thrive to new heights you never thought possible.

Regardless of how you got here and where you'd like your journey as a mother to lead you, here's a prayer, written anonymously, that fits perfectly into where you are *right now*. Let this be your guiding light as you step onto a new path of greater health, greater happiness, and greater fulfillment.

Today may there be peace within. May you trust that you are exactly where you are meant to be. May you not forget the infinite possibilities that are born of faith in yourself and others. May you use the gifts that you have received, and pass on the love that has been given to you. May you be content with yourself just the way you are. Let this knowledge settle into your bones, and allow your soul the freedom to sing, dance, praise, and love. It is there for each and every one of us.

—ANONYMOUS

Chapter 1

Fertility and the Path to Conscious Conception

If you want to have a baby, all you have to do is have sex when you're ovulating and bam! You're pregnant...right? Well, not always. We're not all blessed with especially fertile bodies, and for many women it can take months or even years to conceive. Sometimes it never happens, no matter how much we want it or how hard we're willing to work for it. Conceiving a child can be difficult. It's not a punishment to have to work harder for it, and it's not a free pass not to have to. As women, we're taught to believe that it is our birthright to have a child if we wish to have one, and when we find it difficult to get pregnant, it's easy for feelings of inadequacy and guilt to creep in. We feel like there's something wrong with us as women, and we worry that there's something we're doing wrong that's making us unworthy or incapable of bearing a child.

Many women get it in their heads that life would be incomplete without having a child. We see our friends having babies without even trying to and we feel left out of the loop, like we're not measuring up to the expectations we ourselves have set. Those expectations begin to tear away at us, and the stress we endure as a result can hamper our chances of conceiving even further. Though the ways in which stress inhibits the body's ability to conceive is little understood, research shows there is indeed a

5

correlation. According to a study sponsored by the Eunice Kennedy Shriver National Institute of Child Health and Human Development and published in the *Oxford Journal of Human Reproduction*, high stress levels can more than double a woman's risk of infertility.[1] One young lady who is friends with one of your authors here was only able to get pregnant (both times) when she was on vacation. Why is that, do you suppose? Perhaps the stress and the cloudiness of her mind during any other time made conception more difficult, not because her body was unable to conceive but because her mind did not allow her body to even get to do its part. Our minds are powerful tools that can either do us in or do us justice. It takes effort, but if you want to create the clearest path possible to increase your chances of conception, you'll need to take conscious steps to keep your stress levels at a minimum.

There's a proverb that describes an elderly man telling his grandson, "My son, there is a battle between two wolves inside us all. One is Evil. It is anger, jealousy, greed, resentment, inferiority, lies, and ego. The other is Good. It is joy, peace, love, hope, humility, kindness, empathy, and truth." The boy thought about it, and asked, "Grandfather, which wolf wins?"

The old man quietly replied, "The one you feed."

You must guard against your own "wolves"—those thoughts and feelings that do not serve the purpose of bringing to you a healthy child. Anxiety creates spiritual clutter. Instead, strive to create a sacred passage in your soul, clear of fear, clear of doubt, and illuminated by the light of your spirit. Keep an open mind and don't let fear crowd the pathway. Trust the way, and trust that the perfect child will find its way into your heart one way or another. If you are unable to get pregnant and you desperately want a baby, please consider adoption. There are so many deserving children out there who need a great home. It's the most sacred honor in the world to have a soul choose you to be its parent, and this is true whether or not that child comes through your physical body.

---

1. C. D. Lynch, et al., "Preconception Stress Increases the Risk of Infertility," *Oxford Journal of Human Reproduction* (March 23, 2014), doi:10.1093/humrep/deu032.

Sometimes, all it takes to make it happen is just to step back, clear your head, let go of expectations, and allow whatever will be to be.

When you're trying to get pregnant, it's so easy to get caught up in all the calculations, tracking temperatures, marking dates on the calendar, saving sperm for that ideal moment when it has the best chance of making a baby. This can make sex seem more like a science experiment than an expression of intimacy. When trying to get pregnant becomes a chore, that's when it's time to step back and reevaluate. There is a reason that people get pregnant after adopting a child or after deciding that they are just fine not having a baby after all. They have finally found happiness, which then enables the body's natural rhythm to come forth. In many cases, the body is able to conceive, but stress and other factors can inhibit that ability.

So try to let go of rigid timelines and work instead on making yourself the best you possible. With less stress, a positive outlook, and a balanced emotional state, you'll have the best chance of clearing the path for a child to come to you. You will be able to create a sacred vessel within your soul, opening the way for a special child to choose you to be its very own parent, whether that child finds its way to you through your own body, through adoption, or through other means.

Creating the Way

There are so many things out there that promise to help increase fertility. Women have turned to exercise, acupuncture, massage therapy, chiropractic care, alternative health methods, estrogen, body creams, and so much more in hopes of finding the right formula for creating a child. Some research shows that exercising thirty minutes a day, three days a week, can increase your fertility levels, while other research warns that if you exercise *too* much and start to lose body fat, there's a chance of actually *decreasing* fertility, as the body's natural fat is needed to keep estrogen levels in balance. The role of acupuncture in increasing fertility has also been studied, as the practice is believed to improve circulation to the ovaries and uterus, which makes for healthier eggs and a better chance for implantation. You'll even find advice on what foods to eat (like meat and dairy products) and what foods to avoid (like caffeine and alcohol) to support your fertility.

But getting pregnant is not just about eating the right foods and getting the right amount of rest and exercise. It's not about going to a holistic doctor or slathering on strange creams that may or may not have any effect on your fertility. Conception is so much more than that. Conception can be the conscious creation of a brand-new life, born out of an honest desire to express and share love. You must prepare your spiritual body to become a vessel into which a soul can choose to enter. This is what is meant by conscious conception: you *want* this, you are choosing to be a mother, you are aware of and taking care of your own health inside and out, and you are creating the best, clearest route possible through which a precious child can come to you.

The path to motherhood will be different for each person, of course. But there are a few ideas to keep in mind that will increase the potential for conscious conception:

- You must stay positive and open to conceive. It's not the deciding factor by any means, but maintaining a positive, loving attitude and being flexible in your expectations will increase your chances for success.
- Be healthy, be mindful, and be present to the process. Know that you are exactly where you are meant to be today, and trust that. If you want to have a child, trust that you will have the child that you are meant to have in this life. Trust in whatever roads may lead you to this, and be as open as you can to all the options and possibilities.
- Know yourself and how far you are willing to go to conceive. Adoption, in vitro fertilization, and fertility therapy are not choices everyone is comfortable making. Defining the limits of how far you are willing to go to have a child will help ease the stress caused by a do-or-die attitude that puts pregnancy goals above all others.

Fertility Charms and Symbols
from Around the World

In China, bamboo in the bedroom is believed to boost fertility, while keeping your home's front entrance clean and clear will help relieve barrenness. In Mali, wearing a necklace made of shells is believed to increase one's fertility. In Celtic culture, women who hoped for babies would make a string of hazelnuts that could be hung in the home or worn around the neck as a powerful fertility charm.

Around the world, women have hoped and prayed to be blessed with babies. These prayers have taken many forms, and often additional magickal charms or symbols are used to accompany the prayer and to help fortify the faith and belief of the petitioner. From lucky fruits to lucky animals, fertility charms are as diverse as they are abundant. You might consider giving some of these age-old charms a try. If nothing else, you'll be reminded that you are not alone; many women all over the planet want desperately to be fertile and are ready to try just about anything they can to boost their luck in this endeavor. Although these charms are intended to increase fertility, they can be adapted easily to help bring to you a child through alternative channels such as adoption.

Pomegranates

With their numerous seeds and round appearance, pomegranates have been recognized as a powerful symbol of fertility by many cultures around the world. In ancient Greece, pomegranates were associated with Demeter, a fertility goddess; with Persephone, Demeter's daughter; and with Hera, the goddess of marriage. The fruits were often given as wedding gifts to help encourage lust and/or an abundance of children.[2] In China, pomegranates were placed on the bridal bed along with other fertility symbols in order to help bring children to a newly married couple.[3] In Latin America and other places where Santeria is practiced, pomegranates take a prominent role in certain fertility rites. One such

---

2. Laurence M. V. Totelin, *Hippocratic Recipes: Oral and Written Transmission of Pharmacological Knowledge in Fifth- And Fourth-Century Greece* (Leiden: Brill), 208–209.

3. "Chinese Marriage Charms," Primal Trek, http://primaltrek.com/marriage.html.

ritual requires the woman to write her name on a piece of paper and to place that paper between two halves of a pomegranate. Yemaya, a Yoruban moon goddess, is then petitioned to help make the woman fertile, just like the fruit.[4] Here's a ritual to use if you'd like to try your own pomegranate fertility magick.

Pomegranate Fertility Rite

For this ritual, you will need a pomegranate, a small piece of paper, a pen with blue ink, a knife, and a couple of teaspoons of honey. Begin about three nights prior to the full moon. While thinking of your desire for a child, rub the pomegranate over your belly, then rub it over your bedding or wherever you usually make love. Place the pomegranate under or near the bed or other special place and leave it there until the night of the full moon. Along with the paper, pen, knife, and honey, take the pomegranate outside under the moonlight. Carefully cut the pomegranate in half, and examine the many seeds inside as you think of the children you would like to have. Write your name on the piece of paper followed by the words "is as fertile as this fruit!" Cover the cut sides of the two pomegranate halves with honey as you think of what a sweet blessing a child would be. Place the paper on top of the honey and seal the pomegranate back together so that the paper is sandwiched between the two halves. If you like, say the following words to help strengthen and fortify your intentions:

Mother moon, mother moon,
Bless me with a child soon!
Mother moon, mother moon,
Place a seed within my womb!
Just like this fruit with many seeds,
My womb with child, filled will be!

You might choose to leave the pomegranate tucked in a tree under the moonlight, bury it in the earth, or toss it into a body of water.

---

4. Melissa Meyer, *Thicker Than Water: The Origins of Blood as Symbol and Ritual* (New York: Routledge, 2005), 11.

Coconuts

In Bengal, the milk from a green coconut that had been blessed by a holy person was considered to be a powerful potion to boost fertility.[5] In India, a special vase known as the Purna-Kalasha is used in many fertility rites. Filled with water, topped with a coconut, and crowned with a ring of mango leaves, the Purna-Kalasha represents the fertile womb.[6] The coconut is also associated with fertility in Sri Lanka. One custom practiced at weddings is to split a coconut at the feet of a newly married couple. If the two halves of the coconut land meaty side up, it's taken as an omen of fertility and good fortune.[7] If you want to try some coconut magick yourself, here's a fertility spell that employs coconuts as a main ingredient.

COCONUT FERTILITY RITE

You'll need one whole coconut, some additional coconut milk, an earthen pot, some water, and a handful of dried beans. Begin by placing the earthen pot in front of you. Think of this pot as representing your own womb, or as representing the space in your life that you hope to fill with a new child. Pour water into the pot until it's a little over halfway full. Next, rub the coconut milk all over your belly, moving your hand in a clockwise circle. Think of the fertility-boosting properties of the coconut as you do so. Splash some of the coconut milk into the water-filled pot as well. Next, pick up the beans one by one and cast them into the water, making a wish regarding the welfare of your future child as you do so. For instance, one bean might be for brilliance, while another bean symbolizes a wish for beauty. Finally, place the whole coconut in the pot, visualizing as you do so that it is not a coconut being put into a pot, but a child that is being placed in the womb. Place both hands on

---

5. Pradyot Kumar Maity, *Human Fertility Cults and Rituals of Bengal: A Comparative Study* (New Delhi: Abhinav Publications, 1989), 47.

6. Devdutt Pattanaik, *The Goddess in India: The Five Faces of the Eternal Feminine* (Rochester, VT: Inner Traditions, 2000), 54.

7. "Traditional Sri Lankan Buddhist Wedding Customs," Wedding Things, http://weddingthings.lk/83-articles/latest-news/72-traditional-sri-lankan-buddhist-wedding-customs.

your belly and express clearly in your own words your desire for a child. Visit the pot every day (freshening it when necessary) and repeat your intentions until your wish for a child is fulfilled.

Animal Symbols

Animal symbols have also been employed by many people around the world in hopes of increasing the chances of getting pregnant and having a baby. In many cultures, bulls are associated with male virility and cows are associated with female fertility. In China, fish and elephants are associated with fertility, while frogs have received similar acclaim in South America, Central America, Italy, and Egypt. Rabbits, with their reputation for prolific breeding, are widely revered as symbols of fertility in England, the United States, and many other places.

Try incorporating some fertility-boosting animal symbols into your life and see if it helps your chances of conception. Small stone carvings of these animals might be used as totems to be placed on the altar or near the bed, or you might find a special piece of jewelry to wear that depicts your chosen animal. Fertility-boosting animal symbols might also be featured in fabric motifs for intimate apparel or bedroom décor to help create an atmosphere of faith, fun, and magick as you attempt to conceive. If you have access to the real-life versions of any of the animal symbols described here, take time to observe the animal as you envision yourself sharing the animal's fertile attributes.

Fertility Altar

If you're trying to conceive, you might enjoy creating your own fertility altar, a special place to set intentions, pray, meditate, contemplate, and just clear your head when needed. Your fertility altar could be a coffee table or end table, a nightstand, the top of a dresser, or the top of a shelf. Just make sure the space is clean and free of clutter before you begin creating your sacred altar space.

To get started, cover the surface of your altar with an attractive cloth. Blue and green are colors traditionally associated with fertility, so you might want to choose a cloth in one of those shades. Next, decorate your altar with symbols of fertility. You might incorporate big-bellied goddess statues, baby bottles and baby booties, fruits such as pomegranates or co-conuts, flowers, shells, statues of frogs or rabbits, pictures of children and mothers, or other fertility symbols and motifs.

Spend time at your fertility altar each day. Take some good, deep breaths to center your thoughts, then imagine yourself happily pregnant as you gaze at the images you've placed on the altar. Visualize yourself holding your child to come, and let the love in your heart flow toward the altar. If you like, say a short prayer or an affirmation expressing your desire and your belief in your ability to become a mother.

Keep the Faith and Trust the Way

As you explore different options and strategies along the path to moth-erhood, try to keep an open mind and an open heart. It may take a while, or it may happen sooner than you expect, but if you keep hoping, keep trying, and trust that the path to parenthood will present itself one way or another, a child is bound to find its way into your heart and into your arms. Just don't let the potential challenges and setbacks block the light of your best and brightest intentions.

Chapter 2

You're Pregnant!
Now What?

Who knew that peeing on a stick could bring so much bewilderment so quickly? In one or two lines, your entire life changes forever. You are pregnant. In a flash, an elephant enters the room, and you may even imagine that elephant wearing knitted booties and a matching hat! Your wildest imaginations begin to rumble and explode all within a matter of minutes—sheer excitement mixed with sheer terror in varying proportions, all falling in on you in the form of giant, crashing waves. You begin to realize that whatever habits you were hoping to kick before you got pregnant must now be left behind with an urgency born of absolute necessity, and there is simply no turning back. You try to figure out instantly how to become a better version of yourself. It's time to clean up, like yesterday. It's time to get motivated, get activated, and get situated, because a baby is coming!

It's time to buy and gather baby equipment, set up a nursery, baby-proof your home, get maternity clothes, give up unhealthy habits, learn how to care for an infant, figure out how to be a good parent, and prepare yourself physically, emotionally, and spiritually for giving birth, all while dealing with fluctuating hormones and rising discomfort—oh, and you have just nine months, if you're lucky, to do all this. Forty weeks used to seem like a long time, but once you're pregnant, you realize it's a relatively short time to get everything together for a completely life-changing event. Pregnancy is certainly one of the most overwhelming and exhilarating experiences on earth, as potentially terrifying as it is terrific.

Conscious Conception vs. the "Accidental" Baby

Each woman's perspective on motherhood is unique, and it's important to acknowledge your own genuine feelings toward your pregnancy. Some of us want it, some of us don't want it, and some of us have mixed emotions about it. All these feelings are entirely natural. Despite its tiny size, a baby is a big deal.

Many women end up pregnant without planning to be. We know perfectly well where babies come from, yet accidents and temporary slip-ups in the sensibility department do happen. An unexpected and unplanned pregnancy can bring with it enormous fear and overwhelming stress. Perhaps a baby was something you thought about having much later but not right now, not when you've got so much going on already. It's only natural to feel that way if you're not ready to have a child, but on the other hand, no one is ever *really* 100 percent ready to have a child, as there is no predicting or anticipating the potential challenges and joys that lie ahead.

For other women, pregnancy is immediately recognized as a blessing—at least, until all the hormones and body aches kick in. Perhaps you planned, and waited, and at last deemed it the right time to proceed with having a baby. Perhaps you were able to conceive right away, or perhaps it took a lot of struggling and loss before you succeeded in getting pregnant. The start of the journey to motherhood may be a rocky slope or a slippery slide, and our attitudes about the adventures to come play a huge role in determining just how unpleasant or how enjoyable the experience is.

Whether it's something you planned for and maybe even struggled for or it's something that hit you upside the head like a brick out of nowhere, you're here, expecting a child, right now, and you want to make the most of it. Acknowledge your deepest feelings about having a baby, the negatives as well as the positives. We are all afraid of being pregnant. In fact, you would be a little bit out of touch with reality *not* to have fears when you find out you are pregnant. As an individual, you are entitled to experience any emotions that flow through you, and it's essential to acknowledge these feelings so you can let go of the ones that no longer serve you in your role as a mother. In this early stage of pregnancy, take some time to yourself to think, to hope, to wonder, and to contemplate. Take some time to comfort yourself, to let yourself know that whatever you're feeling right now is okay and will continue to be okay.

Journey into Motherhood Meditation and Ritual

Try this meditation and ritual to help yourself get grounded, centered, and ready for the adventures ahead. Find somewhere quiet and comfortable, and get yourself situated. You'll need a small twig and a dried bean or other seed for this activity; just set them to the side for now. Take some deep breaths until you feel calmer and more relaxed.

Once you're in a peaceful mental state, get in touch with your true feelings about motherhood. How do you feel, honestly, about the journey to come? What are your fears? What are your hopes? What aspects of yourself will serve you well as a mother, and what aspects of your personality or lifestyle will need adjusting? Take time to grieve, if you like, for the life you are losing, and then take equal time to celebrate the new life that is just beginning.

When you're ready, hold the small twig in your hand and think about all the negative feelings, fears, or aspects of your current life that you are ready and willing to put behind you. Think about each one in turn as you hold the twig firmly in your hand, and let the energy of your thoughts flow into the wood. When you're ready to let these feelings and behaviors go, bury the twig, break it up into smaller pieces, or send it floating down a stream or river as you think about how you're ready to move forward.

Now hold the bean or other seed in your hand. Think about everything good you have to offer as a mother. Imagine the joys you will experience and feel the love in your heart that you will share with your child. Let these feelings fill your being and notice how your mood changes. When you're ready, plant the bean or seed. Water it regularly so it will grow in the earth as your child grows within your womb.

To Tell or Not to Tell

The first thing to do if you suspect you're pregnant is to visit a doctor to confirm the pregnancy and begin your care. But beyond your doctor, who should you tell? Do you call every one of your friends right away to tell them the news? Or do you wait until the end of the first trimester or later before you spill the beans?

There are pros and cons to each choice, and what's right for you will likely depend a lot on personal circumstance and past experience. Are your friends and relatives likely to be supportive or critical? Have you had miscarriages in the past, or is this your first pregnancy? If it's your first pregnancy and you're thrilled about it, it will be very difficult to keep yourself from sharing this most exciting news with your dearest family and friends, but all the same, consider the choice carefully, as it is yours to make. On the one hand, it's nice to have others with whom to share your feelings. But on the other hand, once your news is out, oh my, does the flood of unsolicited advice pour in! Opinions run high and fast right out of the gate when it comes to making babies, so brace yourself because they are coming. Immediately people expect for you to have everything in place, to have a plan, and to know all the precise details of your very new pregnancy.

"When are you due, and what are your birthing plans?" That's usually the first thing out, followed by, "I need to introduce you to my coach/doula/midwife/dance teacher/yoga teacher." Very quickly your very personal pregnancy becomes everyone's interest. You get bombarded with horror stories of someone who knew someone. You get overloaded with questions and advice. Everyone seems to know what it is that you need to do, including what you should eat, what activities you should avoid, and what doctor you should choose. This can make your exciting news go from thrilling to scary to downright bothersome very quickly, if you let it.

It's important to have your support systems in place, but at the same time, there is an equally great need to be able to have the space and trust from your friends and family to navigate your body and the space you are in during this time in your own special way. As you will learn during this process, no one is going to approve of every choice you make from start to finish, so beyond following your doctor's advice, trust your instincts and do what you feel is best for you. Whom you choose to share your news with and when depends on your own readiness to face the flood of advice that's bound to come as a result. You may want to consider telling only the people with whom you'd feel comfortable sharing less fortunate news. Honor this choice of yours completely, and choose who you tell with care, based on your own personal feelings. There is absolutely no right or wrong answer to this question.

Setting Boundaries

Because of all the unsolicited advice and opinions that come with pregnancy, it's of the utmost importance to set boundaries for you and your body very early on. There is a very loving way to set boundaries you feel comfortable with and still allow others to share in your joy without overstepping their limits with you from the start. Understand that the reason people usually get their feelings hurt when you reject their advice is not because they hate what you've said, but because the way in which you speak the words can cause feelings of rejection or suspicions of ingratitude. Be firm, but be more loving in tone. Love will carry you much further than will arguments and drama.

Everyone who is trying to offer something to you is doing so because they love you and want you to have the best pregnancy possible. It might be annoying, and some folks definitely do need a few etiquette lessons, but all the same, their hearts are probably in the right place. Try to recognize where others are coming from when they're offering you advice or telling you what to do and what not to do, even if you disagree completely. Try to respond to unwanted opinions in a way that lets people know that you do see where they are coming from and you do love them for it. Then calmly share your own boundaries, perhaps explaining that you are trying to surround yourself with positivity during this very sacred and sensitive time and that you will be making critical decisions on your own time frame based on your own (and your doctor's) best judgment.

An extra little trick you can use to help shield yourself from unwanted energies coming from others is to draw a protective shielding symbol on your belly. You can use a lip liner, eyeliner, or nontoxic marker to create your magickal belly shield. Just be aware that the symbol could potentially rub off on your clothes and stain them, so choose your writing utensil and fashions with care when you try this one. You might draw a pentacle shape or a peace sign. Envision a protective aura emanating out from the symbol to envelop your belly and all the rest of you in an impenetrable shield of loving light. You might also choose to carry with you a piece of hematite or jet, as these stones will help absorb any negative energy headed your way. Carrying a mirror can also help; consider wearing a small one on a necklace to help reflect back any unwanted energies.

Anxiety During Pregnancy

As a mom-to-be, it's completely natural to be anxious during your entire pregnancy. There's so much pressure to do everything you possibly can for your growing baby. Don't make yourself feel too guilty if you're not perfect. In an ideal world, you would juice green drinks every morning, take your prenatal vitamins, and eat five to six small meals every day so your blood sugar stays balanced and you avoid cravings. You would not miss a single doctor appointment. You would exercise daily and meditate often. You would immediately put your growing baby first with every action and decision you make. And if after you saw that very first plus sign you managed to be doing all these things and more, then you would truly be a rock star. Then there are the rest of us—the ones who *want* to do it all right, and do it all right from the start, but who every now and then fall short of the ideal.

Taking good care of yourself and your baby during pregnancy is important; you already know that. Do your best, strive for improvement, and don't let guilt leave you mired in failure. If you have any seriously dangerous behaviors you are trying to manage, such as any eating disorders, severe anxiety disorders, mental disorders, or addictions, don't try to go it alone. Get yourself the help and support you need by talking to a licensed health care practitioner.

Fear is a common feeling during pregnancy. Whatever your biggest pregnancy fears are, do whatever you can in your power to address those first and foremost so you can get back to the business of enjoying this special time in your life. If you're afraid of not having a healthy baby, consider taking any relevant tests that are offered so you can have peace of mind. Be proactive in your pregnancy. If you're constantly worrying about what might go wrong, do whatever you need to do to put your mind at ease. Take that folic acid, especially in the first trimester. If you're drinking or smoking, get some help and stop right away. If you're doing your best to keep your body and your baby healthy, it's a lot easier to allow yourself to relax and think positive.

Essential Oils During Pregnancy

According to Roz Zollinger, owner, aromatherapist, and instructor at the Heal Center (www.healcenteratlanta.com) in Atlanta, Georgia, "One has to be very careful when choosing essential oils to be applied topically (and never internally) to an expectant mom." Some essential oils can be overly stimulating to the nervous system and can potentially trigger uterine contractions. Zollinger advises against using any stimulating essential oils during pregnancy.

Here are Roz Zollinger's lists of some of the top essential oils that should absolutely be *avoided* if you're expecting, and those that can be used safely on the skin. Please note that these are not exhaustive lists. There are many essential oils that have not been thoroughly researched, and their medical benefits and/or risks have not been fully determined. If you're unsure about a particular oil, please consult your doctor or another qualified practitioner. The oils discussed in this book are intended for external use only. The internal use of essential oils is not recommended without the close guidance, supervision, and recommendation of a medical doctor or other qualified health care practitioner.

Top Essential Oils to Avoid During Pregnancy—DO NOT USE!
Bay laurel
Birch
Cajeput

Cinnamon

Clary sage

Clove

Eucalyptus

Ginger

Juniper berry

Lemongrass

Nutmeg

Pennyroyal

Peppermint

Rosemary

Sage

Spanish sage

Tarragon

Thyme

White sage

Wintergreen

Essential Oils That May Be Safely Used Topically During Pregnancy

To use, dilute 1 to 3 drops of essential oil in 1 ounce of a carrier oil, such as sweet almond, jojoba, or organic grapeseed.

Bergamot

Blue tansy

Blue/German chamomile

Cypress

Frankincense

Geranium

Helichrysum/Everlasting/Immortelle

Himalayan cedar

Jasmine

Lavender

Marjoram

Myrrh

Neroli/bitter orange

Roman/English chamomile
Rose
Spikenard
Ylang-ylang

In later chapters, we'll offer more ideas for safe ways to use essential oils during pregnancy, but be sure to stick with these basic guidelines right from the start.

Massage During Pregnancy

Massage is not something just for the rich and famous, and when you get pregnant, you may desperately crave the relief that a full-body massage can provide. There are wonderful ways to cut costs and still get a fabulous massage. Local massage schools usually charge a very reasonable price. If you have health insurance, you may be able to get your massage covered; just check with your insurance provider. Wherever you choose to get a massage, if you choose to get one, it's up to you to guard your body.

First and foremost, do not get a massage during the first trimester of your pregnancy. It's believed that there are several points on the body that, if stimulated through massage or direct pressure, can stimulate uterine contractions. The risk is believed to be higher early on. These same points on the body are sometimes employed very late in pregnancy to help stimulate labor. It's important for you to be aware of, and in charge of, these places on your body. Here is a list—courtesy of Claire Marie Miller, fertility, prenatal, and postnatal massage expert and teacher (www.clairemariemiller.com)—of the points on the body that should not be touched during pregnancy:

- The inner ankle—between the heel and the ankle bone
- Spleen 6 point—located about three centimeters above the ankle bone on the inside of the leg

- Hoku point—located on the hand and the foot; it's the soft webbing between the thumb and the first finger, and the webbing between the big toe and first toe, where it is soft
- Gallbladder 21 point—located in the meaty part of the trapezius muscle on the top of each shoulder
- The sacral dimples—located on the lower back

Some practitioners also caution against touching the Kidney 1 point located on the bottom of the foot, in the upper middle of the foot just below the pads.

You might wonder just how a full-body massage is possible, what with a quickly expanding belly and all. Many therapists will offer you the choice of lying on your side or using a pregnancy pillow that has a little hole cut out at the belly to enable you to lie flat on your stomach. Try both options and see which you prefer.

Setting Intentions

Let's get back to the most important part of all this…you are pregnant. Everything has changed. Time is counted by the week, and it's ticking by quickly. You now view things with the mindset of "we" and not "me." You think before you eat, drink, or act. You double-check the resources to see if you can safely eat this meal, or drink this beverage, or engage in a particular activity. You try to do your very best to protect what is now inside you to help create the greatest pregnancy and spiritual/physical birth possible. You put all your energy and willpower into preparing for the arrival of this special child you created. It's extremely easy to lose yourself in this process, especially with all the discomforts and physical changes that pregnancy brings.

In this first three months (first trimester) of being pregnant, you are wiped out. Absolutely wiped out. You feel exhausted, and your breasts are sore and swollen. As one doctor puts it, the boob fairy has come to visit, and ouch! These first twelve weeks can be very stressful. Since this is the time when your sweet baby's brain is rapidly developing, you want to do everything you can to get through this most fragile stage of pregnancy. You want to stay as positive as you can, which isn't very easy to do when you're feeling awful. Consciously setting your intentions can be a huge help in making it through this potentially stressful period as smoothly and positively as possible.

Now is the time to begin the process of setting your intentions, aligning your mind, body, and spirit to guide you through this most sacred and magickal experience. Now is the time to turn away from your fears and turn instead toward the guiding light of Spirit for strength and will. Try this. Start your mornings by setting your intentions for the day. You can do this while you're still lying in bed when you first awaken, or you can wait until you're up and alert. Just make sure you're comfortable and that the space you're in is free from distractions. Then decide consciously what sort of attitude you will strive to maintain throughout the day, and imagine the experiences you would like to have. What do you wish to be surrounded by today? Happiness? Love? Peace? Wisdom? Envision yourself enveloped in an orb of glowing energy made of love, joy, or whatever strikes your fancy. Stay in that space for a moment, and let your mind and body relax completely. Place your hands on your belly and envision your child growing healthy and strong. If you like, say some words of intention or a prayer for your baby's well-being while you're still there in that relaxed space. Take your intentions and good feelings with you as you begin the rest of the day, and try to hold on to them for as long as possible. If you end up getting stressed-out during the day and you catch yourself slipping into an unpleasant mental state, remember the intentions you set that morning and reaffirm those goals to bring yourself back to center.

The most important thing you can be doing during this time is to stay positive and focused on you, your health, your baby, and your baby's health. The only way you can do that is by consciously deciding to do so, then setting your intentions for how you want to experience pregnancy and sticking to them as best you can. This is the most important thing that you have going on in your life right now. Be thankful and be mindful. It can certainly become very overwhelming, but you can always come back to center by remembering your intentions.

Here's a prayer you can use to help guide your intentions in the highest, most positive direction. It can be addressed to a deity of your choice, to your own higher self, or to the universe in general.

Great Goddess/God/Creator/Great Spirit/Maker of Breath and Giver of Life,

I come to you today to give thanks and ask for your help and support in creating within me a strong, healthy child who will bless this home and our lives. I ask that you guide me to do the best I can during this pregnancy to honor the things that bring health, vitality, and peace of mind and to turn away from the things that are not for the greatest good and highest joy of this amazing spirit growing inside me. Please help me to feel good and strong today, and positive in my thoughts and actions. Please help me to create the best vessel in which this baby can grow and thrive. May this baby continue to grow in a healthy way through birth and way beyond!

Embracing the Magick of Motherhood

Keeping in perspective the immense joy and miraculous blessing that is growing inside you will help you not give in too deeply to the less pleasant physical feelings that often accompany pregnancy. We need to acknowledge the body and what it is going through, but giving more attention to the simple miracle that you are now a part of will help you to stay on the path of the higher self and not give in so easily to hormonal spikes.

At this time, you actually have two hearts beating in your body (or maybe even more than that). This is truly a miracle. Your heart beats life into your body, and at the same time there is a whole new heart that has developed within you that is managing to beat life into a whole new being. Place your hands upon your stomach and feel that underneath your hands is a fully functioning heart beating, bones forming, fingers forming, eyelids and eyelashes all growing right now inside your body as you read this. How utterly phenomenal is that? Your child is a part of you, and you are a part of your child. Use this knowledge to guide you through what is sure to be an incredible time in your life. Although your child cannot yet see the world, you can be your unborn child's eyes. Deliver to your child through your blood and emotions the excitement and wonder of what's to come.

Embracing the Magick of You

Each of us has inside us a spectacular light. Call it the light of Spirit, call it divine inspiration, call it a gift—every single person on earth has something special to offer and share with the world. When you become a mother, your focus will naturally shift to your children, and it's important not to lose sight of your own hopes, dreams, and interests along the way. Just because motherhood has become the top priority doesn't mean you must neglect your other talents. In fact, doing so would be doing yourself, your child, and the world a huge disservice.

You have a gift, a shining place within your spirit that will make your greatest dreams come true if you pay attention to it. Feed that light within you; fuel it with creativity and courage, and let it shine brightly for the world to see. Whether it's art, writing, crafts, business, music, healing, helping, or something else entirely that ignites your passions, go for it. Being a mother can get boring and banal if that's all you are, so don't forget to nourish yourself and pursue your non-mommy dreams too. Share your gifts without any reservations or expectations. Be willing to honor that part of yourself, that special light that makes you be *you*, throughout pregnancy and beyond so that you can do the same for your new child.

Chapter 3

~~~∽·ᕼ~~~

Pregnancy Stretches

When you're pregnant, your entire body changes. Your internal organs shift to make more room for the baby, which makes it incredibly uncomfortable just to breathe normally. Everything makes you feel a need to rush to the bathroom, and the fire in your chest and throat only add to the discomfort. These unpleasant sensations are just some of the side effects that come with growing a precious baby. Fortunately, pregnancy need not be such an uncomfortable experience. This is a sacred time in your life and you want to enjoy it. You don't want to let physical discomfort get in the way of embracing how special pregnancy can be, and the good news is, you don't have to.

There are many effective tools you can use to help minimize the unpleasantness and maximize the joyfulness of pregnancy. One such tool is stretching. Stretching our muscles and tendons can relieve discomfort, ease tension, improve flexibility, and lessen both physical and emotional stress. In this chapter, you'll discover some simple stretching and breathing techniques to help keep you comfortable while that special baby in your belly continues to grow.

Each of these exercises can be done throughout all three trimesters of pregnancy (and beyond, for that matter), but you don't need to do every single one in order to gain the benefits. As your body slows down and you find yourself getting more tired as labor approaches, simply pick and choose which stretches you need, and perform them in the position that's the most comfortable for you.

As with any physical exercise program, it's a good idea to ask your doctor for the go-ahead before you begin. For each technique, you'll find a description as well as a photo of our lovely model Colette Short-house taken at Johns Creek Yoga Studio in Johns Creek, Georgia. Read through each technique a couple of times before you try it, and let the photos guide you. These easy-to-learn, gentle exercises will help you gain some much-needed relief during this wonderful yet often uncomfortable time. All you'll need for these simple stretches and breathing techniques is yourself and a small blanket. Fold up the blanket so it makes a little cushion, and sit so your bottom is on the blanket but your legs are not. This position helps the spine elongate to be as straight as possible. Just sitting in this position makes it a little easier to take fuller, deeper breaths.

Setting the Tone with Your Breath

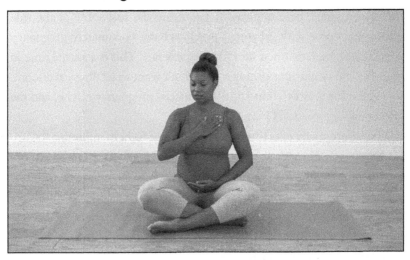

Figure 1: Setting the Tone with Breath

A good way to begin your stretching routine is to set the tone with your breath. Sit with your legs in a modified crisscross position with one leg in front of the other, or if this is not comfortable, bend your knees and open up your legs to help your middle expand. Place one hand on your chest and one hand on your sweet belly. Breathe slow, easy, full breaths, in and out (figure 1). Feel your belly and chest expand. When you're not pregnant, you focus solely on the belly expanding with the breath, and the chest is kept rather still. But with a growing baby quickly taking up so much space inside that belly, you want to fill your stomach, your chest, and even your collarbones up with the air—expanding the lungs fully as you imagine that breath circulating throughout your body. Just be sure to keep your shoulders lowered. If your shoulders lift up, you will only increase the tension in your body, so keep those shoulders down and relaxed. Keep your breathing slow and gentle, bringing a calming, centering energy into your body with each breath. See yourself healthy, radiant, serene, and full of life.

Sunshine Breaths

Next, try this beautiful, easy breathing technique to help lift and lengthen your torso and spine. Starting with the arms down by your sides (figure 2a), inhale and lift the arms up and overhead (figure 2b), breathing through your nose as you do so. On the exhale, lower the arms back down (figure 2c), open your mouth, and exhale through the mouth. This move naturally expands the belly, lungs, diaphragm, chest, and clavicle to give you 100 percent full breathing capacity.

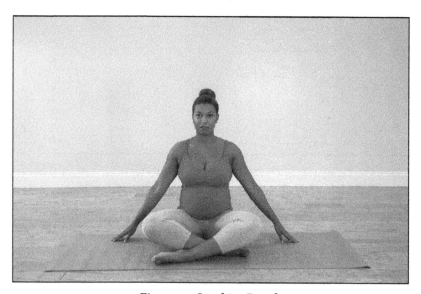

Figure 2a: Sunshine Breath

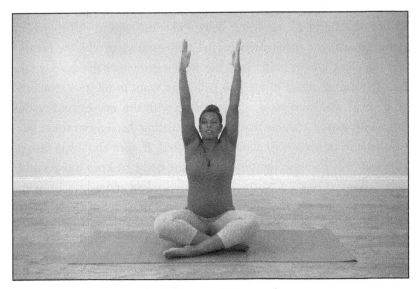

Figure 2b: Sunshine Breath

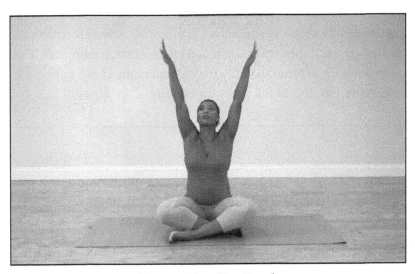

Figure 2c: Sunshine Breath

Sunshine Breathing Visualization: As you inhale and lift your arms
   up and overhead, imagine that you are bringing in the sunlight and
   filling up your entire being with the radiant health, heat, and color
   of the sun. Fill your body with joy and expansion. As you exhale and

bring your arms back down, keep the energy of the sunshine within you, but now mix it with the energy of the earth. Feel that rooting, grounding, available energy combining with these powerful forces of sun and earth. Do this several times. Let your baby feel the perfect blend of the energy they are now in as they grow within the womb, still floating in and out of the ethers and coming in and out of the earth, preparing themselves for life. Bring the sunshine to your child.

Angel Breathing

For the angel breathing technique, sit up straight and clasp your hands together underneath your chin (figure 3a). Exhale all the air in your lungs completely before you proceed. Inhale and keep your hands clasped under the chin, but spread the elbows out wide and lift the chin up and back to point to the ceiling (figure 3b). Exhale and bring the elbows back together (figure 3c) as you slowly lower the chin. You will feel your lungs, chest, and neck all working together to bring beautiful relief from the tightness you may be experiencing. Do this for at least three full rounds.

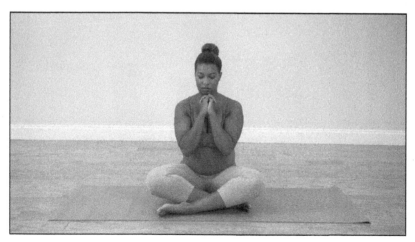

Figure 3a: Angel Breathing

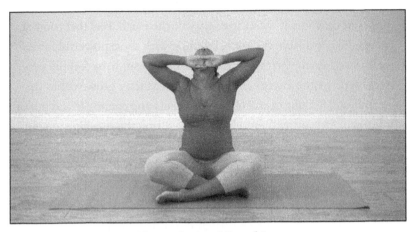

Figure 3b: Angel Breathing

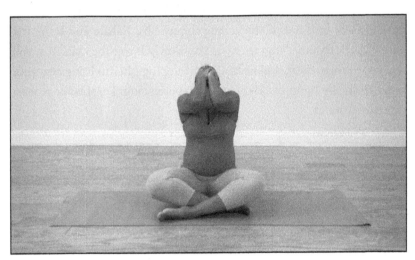

Figure 3c: Angel Breathing

Visualization: Concentrate on your energy being full and light, almost weightless. When you do this angel breath, notice how your entire body fills with oxygen and joy. Visualize a shining, pure, white or golden light filling your whole body. As you exhale, bring the energy back down to the center of your being. Open up your wings as you expand both the elbows and the lungs. Come back to earth as you close up and come down.

Kegels

Kegels are extremely important to do every day during your pregnancy to strengthen the muscles of the pelvic floor. Plus, the stronger your muscles are down there, the better chance you'll have of delivering your baby without tearing the perineum (the tender skin between the genitals and the anus—yeah, super ouch).

Sit with your bottom and feet flat on the floor, your knees bent comfortably. Straighten your spine, and give that middle area some room to breathe. You can place your hands behind you, on your legs, or in prayer position. Do whatever is most comfortable for you. It's easiest to do Kegels when you match the exercise to your breath. Inhale and gently acknowledge that area between the genitals and the anus/perineum, then tighten that area and gently pull it up toward the navel. On the exhale, relax this area. You can actually do Kegel exercises throughout the day in virtually any position, but it's especially easy to get the hang of it from this seated position.

Kegels Visualization: The area of the body in which Kegel exercises are performed is also referred to as the *mula banda* in yoga. It is a very sacred energy space, and by locking it in and pulling it up, we are greatly increasing our energy in this area. This is the location of a magickal place, a place where earth combines with ethereal and brings energy up into the sacred parts of your being. Close your eyes and go deep within to this area and your baby just above this area. Bring the light into your body and into the birth sac. Bring in powerful earth energy, visualizing this energy as a red- or orange-colored light. Blend these powerful energies around your baby. Strengthening the energy in this area helps keep your muscles strong as your baby grows and will also help you push the baby out once it's time for delivery, if you're doing a vaginal birth. Focus your mind on the muscles in this area. Focus on the energy and feel it all moving inward and upward into your being.

The Cat and Cow for Stretching the Spine and Torso

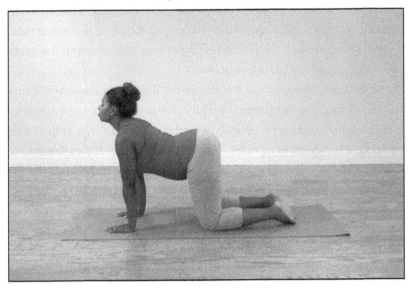

Figure 4a: Cat Pose

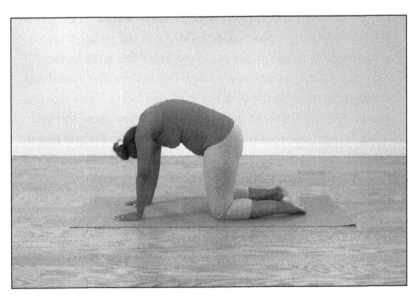

Figure 4b: Cow Pose

For the cat-cow stretch, get up on your hands and knees, placing your knees just under your hips and your hands just under your shoulders. Inhale and drop the pubic bone down toward the ground and lift your chin up to the ceiling, giving a nice arch to the spine. In yoga, this is known as cat pose (figure 4a). Now exhale and round the back as high as you can as you look toward your navel. This is cow pose (figure 4b). Flow between these two poses for at least five rounds. You can also do a standing version of the same stretch (figures 5a and 5b).

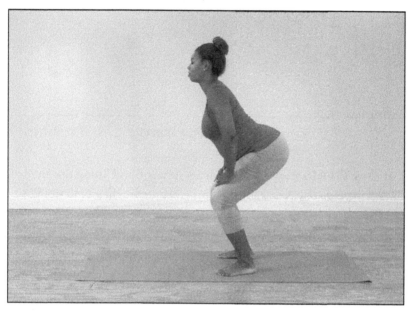

Figure 5a: Cat Pose Standing

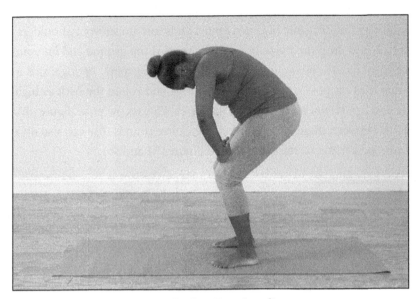

Figure 5b: Cow Pose Standing

Cat-Cow Visualization: When you are inhaling and lifting the chin and the chest up into cat pose, this is the time when your entire heart space expands and lifts to the heavens. Open your heart in this position to the highest vibration of love you can imagine. When you exhale and look toward your growing belly in cow pose, take the love that you just inhaled and now exhale it right down to your little baby.

The Potter's Squat

For this pose, squat as low as you are able. This photo shows a great starting point for this exercise (figure 6), but as you gain practice, see if you can drop your bottom even lower to the ground. It helps to turn your toes out slightly. Keep your palms together for balance and centering. Hold this pose as long as you feel comfortable. It will relieve stress from many parts of the body.

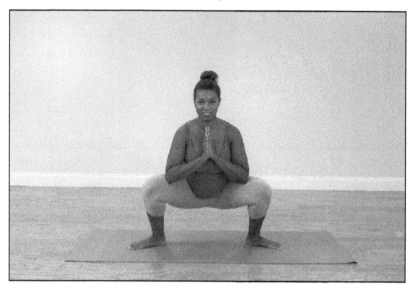

Figure 6: Potter's Squat

Potter's Squat Visualization: Try to sense the energy of the earth beneath you, and pull this energy up into your lower pelvic floor. Imagine a peaceful energy forming between your palms, then bring this energy into your heart. You might visualize it as a soft and serene lavender light. Let this energy radiate from your heart and swirl around your entire being, filling both you and your baby with strength and power.

Torso Stretch

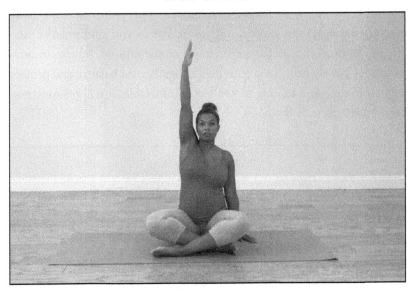

Figure 7a: Torso Stretch

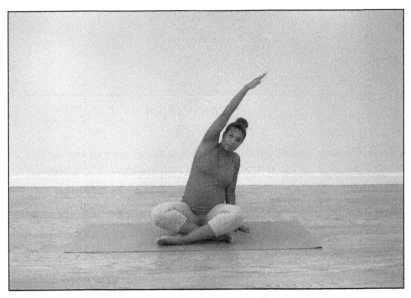

Figure 7b: Torso Stretch

For the torso stretch, bring one arm straight up by the ear and reach up to the ceiling with a nice inhale (figure 7a). On the exhale, bring that arm directly over to the side. Keep the arm next to the ear and feel the sides of your body stretch (figure 7b). Then change sides and repeat. This stretch opens up so much room for you and your growing baby to be able to breathe more comfortably. This is one of the best stretches to use during pregnancy; in fact, you might just want to use it all day long. You can vary this basic stretch by simply turning the head to look up, again continuing to keep the arm close to the ear.

Chest Stretch

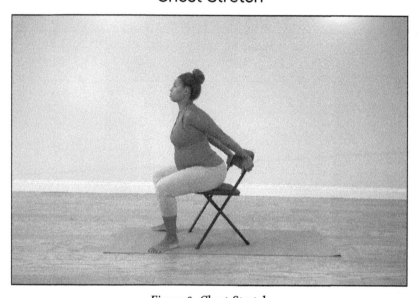

Figure 8: Chest Stretch

For the chest stretch, sit in a chair and place your hands on the back of the chair. Move your chest forward as far as you can until your arms can straighten (figure 8). You can also do this stretch standing, with your hands gripping the inside edges of a doorway. You'll be amazed how good this feels.

Wrist Stretch

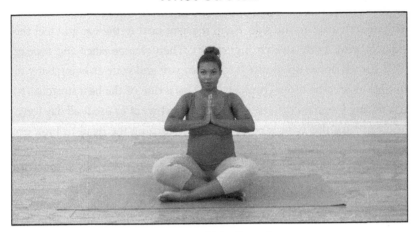

Figure 9a: Wrist Stretch

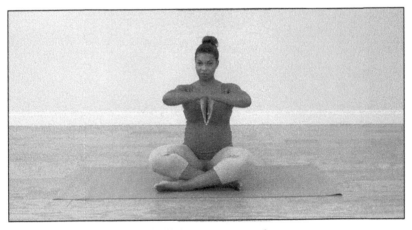

Figure 9b: Wrist Stretch

The joints become more lax during pregnancy, and you may be more prone to stress in the muscles and joints. This can increase your chances of experiencing symptoms common to carpal tunnel syndrome. This simple wrist stretch can help you avoid these issues.

Press both palms together, making sure that you get the base of the hands to touch as best you can. Let the elbows be straight out to the sides (figure 9a). Push the palms of the hands against each other to stretch the wrist muscles as well as the palms themselves. Next, place both hands together but this time with the fingers pointing down and the knuckles of the hands facing each other (figure 9b). See if you are able to drop your elbows below the straight plane to each side. If you can't do it, keep working on it, but don't push too hard.

Butterfly Stretch

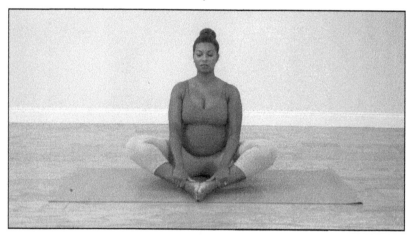

Figure 10a: Butterfly Stretch

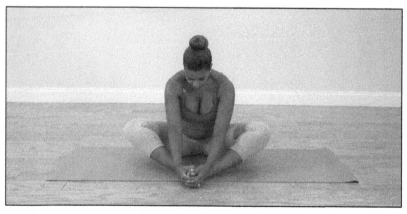

Figure 10b: Butterfly Stretch

For the butterfly stretch, sit with your bottom on the blanket's edge, and gently bring your legs out and touch your feet together (figure 10a). Don't worry about bringing the feet too close to the body. Be gentle with your hips here. Put your feet together and gently bring your body forward into a nice, gentle butterfly stretch (figure 10b).

Seated Forward Bend

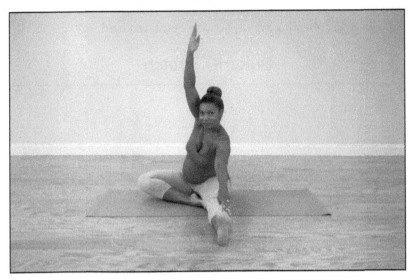

Figure 11a: Seated Forward Bend

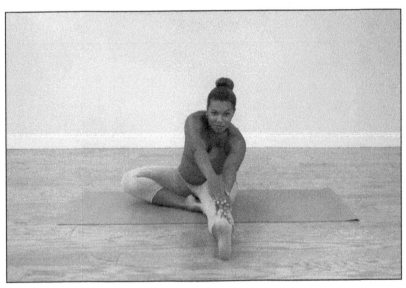

Figure 11b: Seated Forward Bend

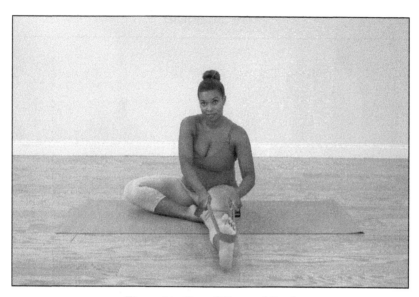

Figure 11c: Seated Forward Bend

For the seated forward bend, begin in butterfly stretch (figure 10a). Then extend one leg straight out and bring your bent leg in a little bit closer to the body. Try to reach out to the extended foot. If your left hand is reaching out to your left foot, stretch your right arm up high to elongate the spine fully (figure 11a). Next, reach with both hands to the extended foot (figure 11b). This really helps to open the hips as well as the hamstrings. Hold each pose for at least five deep breaths. Change sides and repeat. Use a strap or towel around the extended foot if you are not able to comfortably reach the foot yourself (figure 11c).

Next, try extending both legs out in front of you so that your feet are shoulder length apart. You can use a strap or towel to place around your feet if it is not comfortable to reach the feet and bend forward. Or if it is comfortable for you, try to reach your feet and then bend forward. Do not pull your body beyond its limits. This is a stretch to release tension from the lower back and to stretch the hamstrings. There is no need to overdo it. Be gentle.

The Straddle

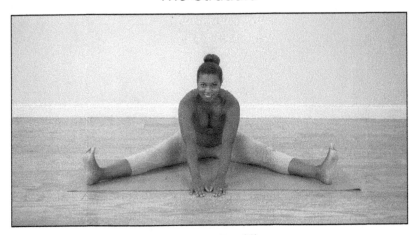

Figure 12a: Straddle

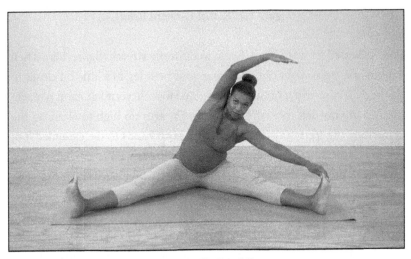

Figure 12b: Straddle

For the straddle, gently bring the legs out wide to the sides (figure 12a). Only go as far as you are able with your legs straight. If you bend your knees, it negates the stretch for the hamstrings. To stretch each side, you can reach out to your feet, you can place one elbow on the thigh, or you can grab your toes while you bring the other arm up and over the ear (figure 12b). Do this on both sides.

Hip Stretch

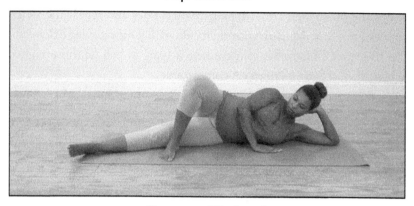

Figure 13a: Hip Stretch

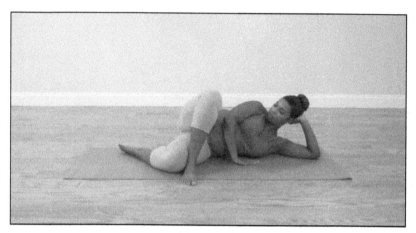

Figure 13b: Hip Stretch

As your pregnancy progresses, more and more hormones are released to help loosen the hips in preparation for childbirth, and the hips can become very achy. This stretch can help relieve a lot of the discomfort. Start by lying on your side. Place your arm in a bent position underneath you to keep your body balanced. Start on your left side with your left leg extended. Bend your right leg and bring the right foot flat on the floor in front of your left leg (figure 13a). The key to increasing this stretch is to take the leg that is extended, in this case the left leg, and bend that knee to move the right leg in closer to your body, thus targeting that upper, outer thigh area (figure 13b). The bent leg that just scooted in is what keeps the other foot from slipping. Switch sides and repeat the same process, this time lying on your right side with your right leg extended. Do this stretch often. You can even do it lying in bed on those nights when you just can't seem to get comfortable.

Seated Lumbar Spinal Twist

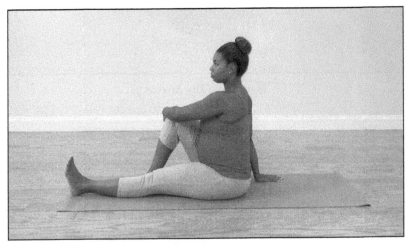

Figure 14a: Seated Lumbar Spinal Twist

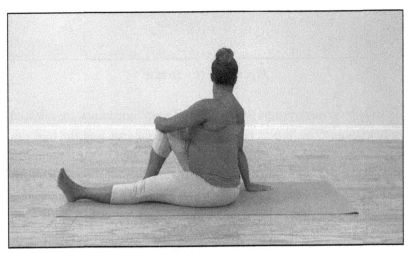

Figure 14b: Seated Lumbar Spinal Twist

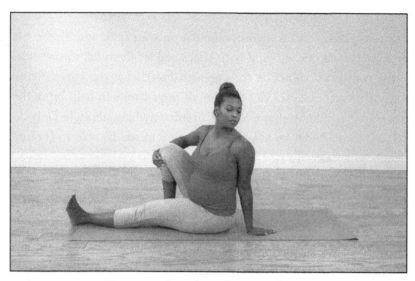

Figure 14c: Seated Lumbar Spinal Twist

For the seated lumbar spinal twist, begin by bending your right knee. Bring your right arm behind you so that it's in line with your spine. Your palm should be flat on the floor for support. Keep your back as straight as possible. Hug your right knee with your left arm and look over your right shoulder (figures 14a and 14b). Next, switch to the other side, bringing your left arm behind you so that it's in line with your spine, your palm again placed flat on the floor. With your right hand, hug your right knee and gently look over your left shoulder (figure 14c). This will help to open the spine and help any stagnant energy release from the lungs.

Gentle Spinal Twist on the Floor

For the spinal twist on the floor, lie flat on your back and extend the arms out to each side. Bend both knees and let them fall to one side. Bring your head to look in the opposite direction as the knees (figure 15). As a variation, you can use one of your hands to help bring the knees over a little bit more. Do not overdo anything, though. Only do what is comfortable for you and allows you to still be able to breathe deeply with ease.

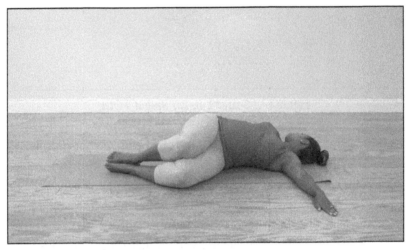

Figure 15: Gentle Spinal Twist on Floor

After-Stretch Cooldown

Seated on your bottom or on your heels in a kneeling position, take time to connect again with your baby after completing these stretches. Place your hands on your tummy and test various hand positions to see what feels best to you, what helps you to connect more with your baby. Think of the love that lives in your heart, and let that loving energy flow directly to your baby as you enjoy several long, slow, relaxing breaths.

End with a nice belly rub. This brings more relief than you may realize. During pregnancy, constipation is common, so much so that most prenatal vitamin supplements come with a stool softener. Rubbing your belly the right way can stimulate the digestive tract and aid digestion.

Starting at the top of your belly, rub in a circular motion, going only clockwise. (Think of your head as twelve o'clock, your left side as three o'clock, your feet as six o'clock, and your right side as nine o'clock.) We go only in this direction because this follows the direction of the colon. Circle from top to left to bottom to right.

Lastly, be sure to lie down and relax if you have time to do so after stretching. In pregnancy, the best way to lie down is on your left side. This is the healthiest and easiest way to nourish both you and the baby. The reason we don't want to lie flat on our backs after twenty weeks is because of the blood flow. There is a very large vein called the inferior vena cava that runs just to the right of the spine. As the uterus grows, it can impede the blood flow back to the heart. This means that less blood makes it back to your heart and the baby's heart. When you lie down, try using a blanket as a pillow for your head, with a body pillow or regular pillow between your knees. Try to relax in that position for about five minutes to allow your muscles and your mind to absorb all the work you just did.

Other Ways to Get Active

In addition to stretching, you might want to try a few other light to moderate physical activities to help you stay in shape and feel great throughout your pregnancy. As always, check with your doctor first. Choose an activity that suits your needs, schedule, and interests. Love dancing? Consider signing up for dance instruction. Love the water? Sign up for a water aerobics class. Is communing with nature your thing? Try to take a short walk outside a few times a week, or daily if you can manage it. Can't leave the house because you're too busy watching children who have already been born and are currently running around like crazy? Try a simple yoga, stretch, or exercise DVD. The possibilities are endless, but the important thing is to pick something, get your doctor's clearance, and then get moving. Your body and your baby will thank you.

Chapter 4

~~~

Embracing Your Inner Mama

Pregnancy and motherhood are both what you make of them. Bringing children into the world and raising those children to the best of your ability can be the most joyous and exciting adventure ever, or it can be an incredible burden, a constant struggle to keep your own head above water while doing the best you can for your kids. As a parent, there are many things beyond your control. You may not have the best financial situation, or the best support system, or a number of other assets that can make parenting a whole lot easier. But you do have control over your own outlook, the way you choose to view the challenges of parenthood and the way you choose to see yourself as a mother. Cultivating positive feelings toward yourself and your baby now, while you're pregnant, can help set you up for greater happiness and success later on when the baby arrives.

In this chapter, you'll explore some ways to connect with and empower your own inner mama, and you'll also learn several techniques you can use to communicate with your baby right now, while they are still growing inside you.

Discovering the Mother Goddess Within

Within every woman, and within every mother, there is a goddess, a spiritual being with tremendous power and infinite potential. Exploring the goddess archetype in its many forms can help you discover and tap into the goddess you truly are, transcending limitations and shining like a star each day. Around the world, mother goddesses abound, an ancient archetype often connected with the earth and the powers of creation. For thousands of years, such goddesses have been petitioned for help with fertility, pregnancy, childbirth, lactation, and other goals particular to mothers and mothers-to-be.

Take a look at this sampling of mother goddesses from around the world, and if anything calls to you, consider studying the archetype further. Is there a goddess who embodies characteristics you would like to reflect in your own life? Is there a goddess who represents just the thing you need right now? In what ways are you like this goddess? In what ways are you different? Observe your feelings and be genuine with your impressions; you might just discover the goddess within you during the process.

Anahit (Armenian): Goddess of healing, birth, fertility, beauty, water, and wisdom. Her symbols are the rose, the dove, gold, and water. Anahit can be called on to help with conception difficulties, protect the womb, ease childbirth, and aid in lactation. Connect with Anahit through dance, music, or offerings of roses or water. You might also wear a special piece of gold-toned jewelry to invoke her energies.

Asase Ya (Ashanti): Goddess of fertility, motherhood, the earth, and the harvest. Having the power to sustain life, Asase Ya is honored in rituals of gratitude following the safe birth and naming of a new child. Her symbols are earth, fields, and the planet Jupiter. Connect with Asase Ya by pouring water or other libations onto the bare earth or by simply enjoying the sights and smells of the soil and plants around you.

Cybele (Phrygian): Goddess of motherhood, fertility, animals, mountains, and the wild earth. Her symbols are unpolished stones and the lioness. Fierce, protective, and powerful, Cybele can be called on to provide extra strength, defense, and energy for mothers and children alike. Connect with Cybele through ecstatic music, drumming, and dancing or by meditating on the lioness totem.

Eileithyia (Minoan): Goddess of childbirth and midwifery. Presiding over the delivery, Eileithyia can be called on to bring on or delay labor and to ensure a child's safe passage into the world. Her symbols are the torch and the cave. Connect to Eileithyia through singing, music, or gazing at a candle flame, or by offering a lock of your hair, a piece of your clothing, or a piece of jewelry such as a necklace.

Hathor (Egyptian): Goddess of childbirth, motherhood, fertility, love, joy, music, and dance. Known as the Mother of Mothers, Hathor can be called on for protection and comfort during childbirth, to help ensure a pleasant and successful pregnancy, and to increase the joy and pleasures of motherhood. Her symbols are cows, drums, sistrums, and mirrors. Connect to her through music making or by gazing into a mirror.

Laima (Baltic): Goddess of luck, fate, happiness, mothers, conception, pregnancy, and childbirth. Her symbols are woven cloth, towels, and baths. Laima can be called on to help with conception, to encourage a safe and speedy delivery, and to brighten your spirits when you're feeling down. Connect with Laima by taking a long, relaxing bath or by bathing the arms or head with a wet washcloth.

Lucina (Roman): Goddess of fertility, childbirth, the moon, and the protection of women. Call on Lucina for help with conception or for protection throughout pregnancy and labor. You can connect with Lucina through offerings of silver coins or through the sharing of feasts. It was believed that by loosening the hair and undoing any knots in your clothing, Lucina would be prompted to remove any hindrances to labor, making for an easy birth. Her symbols are the moon, the ladybug, and the spindle.

Nuakea (Hawaiian): Goddess of milk and lactation. Call on Nuakea to bring milk or for help during the weaning process. Her symbols are breasts and milk. Connect with Nuakea by spilling milk on the earth or by placing your hands on your breasts and calling her name.

Rhea (Greek): Goddess of motherhood, fertility, mountains, and the earth. Gentle and comforting, Rhea can be petitioned to lessen the pains of labor and to bring the mother strength during delivery. Her symbols are the lion, the oak, and the chariot. Connect to Rhea through playing drums, horns, or cymbals, through dancing, through offerings of oak leaves, or through meditating on the lion totem.

Sinivali (Hindu): Goddess of fertility, conception, and childbirth. Call on Sinivali for help with conception or to ease the pain of labor. Her symbols are the cow and the crescent moon. Connect with Sinivali through meditating on the new moon or by wearing a crescent-shaped pendant.

Taweret (Egyptian): Goddess of water, child rearing, birth, care giving, and household protection. Her symbols are the hippopotamus, the lion, the crocodile, the acacia tree, water lilies, and water. Fiercely protective, Taweret can be called on to protect the baby during pregnancy and birth or to guard the family at any time. Connect with Taweret through offerings of water, through ritual bathing or swimming, or by wearing an amulet featuring Taweret's image or that of a hippopotamus, crocodile, or lion.

Xochiquetzal (Aztec): Goddess of pregnancy, childbirth, beauty, pleasure, and textile arts. Strong, beautiful, loving, and youthful, Xochiquetzal can be called on to protect young mothers, ease the pain of childbirth, and improve sexual intimacy between you and your partner. Her symbols are birds, butterflies, and flowers, especially the marigold. Connect with Xochiquetzal by watching birds and listening to their songs, observing butterflies, surrounding yourself with flowers, or engaging in textile arts such as embroidery, weaving, or sewing.

Working with the Mother Goddess

As you can see from the small sampling just given, the mother goddess takes many forms, just as we ordinary, everyday mothers take many forms. There is no one right way to be a mother, and the type of mother you will be is entirely up to you. Working with the mother goddess archetype in a form that calls to you will help you to discover your full potential as a mother, and the steps along the journey will help you to achieve that potential and perhaps even surpass it.

Choose a goddess from the previous list or find another maternal archetype that appeals to you. You might even choose a human mother to be your source of inspiration, someone who exemplifies your personal idea of the ideal mother. Set up a special place in your home to pay homage to this archetype, a space reserved for meditations, prayers, and rituals, or simply to refresh yourself and get inspired. You might include goddess statues and symbols associated with the archetype you've selected. You might include items representing motherhood and the type of mother you want to be.

Each day, go to this special place in your home and spend a few moments thinking about this maternal archetype. Who is this goddess, this cosmic mother? What is she saying to you? What wisdom and skills does she possess that you would like to cultivate? How can you adopt these traits for yourself? Ask and listen. After some minutes in silence, write down any messages or visions that came to you. Write down at least one new thing you noticed about this particular motherly energy. Express your gratitude for the moment and leave a small token of thanks, such as a flower, a cup of water or wine, or some coins.

Animal Totems for Moms

All moms can use a little extra inspiration every now and then, and one place we might not think to look for it is in the animal kingdom. Animal moms have many different styles of parenting, sometimes mirroring our own, sometimes contradicting the way we personally would do things. From all of them, however, we can learn something.

Check out the following mother animal totems and see if anything calls to you. If you find one that you feel is in sync with your personality or that reflects traits you would like to cultivate as a mother, consider making it your personal animal totem, an animal spirit archetype that acts as a special helper and guide. You can wear a piece of jewelry with a pendant featuring your animal of choice; put in your home a photo, statue, stuffed animal, or other symbol of the animal; or carry around a small token representing the animal, such as a small figurine. Meditate on your animal totem whenever you feel you need an extra boost to remind you of your better qualities and to inspire you to achieve your full potential. See yourself as the animal, or imagine the animal walking side by side with you, as a friend and faithful guardian.

Bear: Strength, confidence, and practicality characterize the mother bear totem, encouraging us to make our kids our number-one priority while making the best use of our skills and resources. In the wild, many bears, such as the American black bear, rely on their mothers for food, protection, and education. Nursing her cubs for three months without eating anything herself, the American black bear understands that being a mommy often means making sacrifices. Later, mother bears must teach their cubs hunting skills, how to make a den, and more, all while gathering food and fending off predators. Even with so much to do, they're always ready to answer the beckoning cries of their young. Although they're quite busy, mother bears know the value of rest, so be sure to save some time for extra sleep and relaxation.

Crocodile: Wisdom, ferocity, and awareness characterize the mother crocodile totem. Crocodile mothers guard their nests throughout the incubation period, and they're so in tune with their babies that they can hear their cries even before they hatch. The baby crocodiles make sounds to signal their siblings and their mother that it's time to hatch, and the mother crocodile responds by digging up the eggs and providing assistance. Crocodile mothers transport their young through the water safely by carrying them gently in their massive jaws or by letting them ride on their head or back. Even as the baby crocodiles grow, the mother eagerly fights off predators who would otherwise destroy her young. Ferocious when danger strikes but careful and protective toward her own brood, the crocodile mother reminds us that both strength and gentleness are necessary for successful parenting.

Eagle: Far-seeing and high-flying, the mother eagle totem illustrates the value of attaining a broad-minded yet keenly aware perspective on parenthood. Eagle moms keep a close eye on their young, staying with them in the nest for the first couple of months, then gradually moving to nearby perches to continue overseeing and providing food until the eaglets are able to fly and hunt on their own. Eagle parents share much of the familial responsibility, with both the mom and the dad taking turns hunting, defending the nest, and caring for the young. Soaring high in the sky and traversing great distances quickly, the eagle mother reminds us to take a step back sometimes and see the bigger picture.

Elephant: Commitment and compassion are the trademarks of the mother elephant totem. Nursing their young for up to three years and keeping them close throughout childhood or beyond, elephant mothers are a source of affection, strength, and reliability for their children. Other females in the elephant herd pitch in to help the mother feed and protect her young, illustrating that a community-based approach to child rearing has its merits. The elephant mom reminds us to be dedicated parents committed to our duties and also urges us to accept help when we need it from the people we trust.

Gorilla: Peaceful, protective, and affectionate, the mother gorilla totem encapsulates the idea of nurturing, sustaining love. Mother gorillas sleep with their young, hold them, cuddle them, feed them, teach them, and protect them. For the first two and a half years of life, the young gorilla often travels on its mother's back for safety, observing everything she does and absorbing essential knowledge all while strengthening the mother-baby bond. Gorilla mothers stay close to their babies, slowly acclimating them to more independent living. Patient and compassionate, the gorilla mother teaches us to give our time and energy to our babies and not to be stingy with our shows of affection.

Turtle: Tenacious, methodical, and independent, the mother turtle totem illustrates the value of advanced planning and preparation. After carefully choosing an ideal nesting site, the mother turtle lays her eggs and goes on her merry way, leaving it up to the babies to feed and protect themselves. It might sound heartless to us humans, who hopefully know better than to abandon our babies, but at the same time, the freedom enjoyed by the turtle mother is attractive and reminds us to avoid the urge to hover and micromanage every aspect of our children's development. Our babies, just like turtle babies, have instincts, and they need a reasonable amount of room to grow and explore independently of their parents. Turtle mamas are not always so uninvolved, however. Yellow-bellied sliders have been observed teaching their young how to swim, while Amazonian river turtles have been heard communicating with their hatchlings through vocalizations intended to coax the wee turtles into the water. Turtle moms take their space, but only after they take care of business.

Wolf: Intuitive, intelligent, and family-oriented, the mother wolf totem teaches us to trust our instincts and to value our social and emotional bonds. For the first few weeks after a mother wolf gives birth, she rarely leaves the den, preferring to stay with her pups to provide them with milk, warmth, and protection. As the wolf pups grow, other members of the wolf pack lend their aid to the care and education of the young. Wolf mothers have tremendous endurance and are highly reliant on the rest of the pack, reminding us that even though we can survive independently, we can all use a little help now and then.

Communicating with the Baby inside You

You don't have to wait for your baby to get here before you start being a mama. You're a mama right now, so you might as well embrace it and make the most of this time. There are lots of ways to get acquainted with your baby right now and to express to your child your love and other emotions. We've all seen TV shows where the daddy leans down to the mom's belly to talk to the baby. This might seem silly, but it's important to do. Even though it's extremely loud in the womb, with all the swooshing sounds of blood flowing, the mother's breathing, and a sac of amniotic fluid surrounding them, babies can still hear voices, music, and other sounds well before they are born. Many mothers also report that their babies seem to respond to touches on the belly and to energy work such as Reiki.

Try the following techniques to connect and communicate with the baby inside you. Doing so will awaken your maternal instincts to help you feel more excited, optimistic, and ready for the incredible task of motherhood that lies before you, and it will also help to develop the connection your baby will have to you and your partner.

Hand Placements for Connecting with Baby

There are several hand positions you can use to help you connect to your baby. For the triangle, place your hands at the center of your belly, your thumbs touching at the tips and your other fingers meeting below to create a triangular space in the middle of your hands. Gaze at the little triangle of belly peeking through, and think about the child growing inside you. Can you feel the baby's spirit moving within you? Can you imagine the tiny body wiggling about inside you? Breathe slowly and deeply, drawing powerful earth energies from beneath your feet all the way up through your body and into your little baby.

Another position to try is to place one hand at the top of your belly and the other hand at the bottom, cradling that beautiful round baby bump. Keep your breathing long and slow. Know that the baby can feel everything you are sending to them. Think about your love for this child, the comfort and nurturing you will provide to them. Envision the energy of your thoughts flowing out through your hands and into your belly to reach the baby inside your womb. Trust in the power of intention, and visualize all the loving, glowing, healing light you can imagine wrapping around your baby like a mother's hug. Does your baby have a message for you in response? Pay attention to the thoughts and feelings that come to you at this time.

Another good hand position for connecting with your baby is the side placement. Put one hand on the right side of your belly and one hand on the left side. You can spread your fingers out wide or keep them close together, whichever you prefer. Breathe deeply into the space of your baby. Feel the baby move around inside of you, or if you're not far enough along to feel this yet, imagine those movements. What energies do you feel emanating from your womb? What do you think your baby is feeling right now, thinking right now, doing right now? See your baby in your mind's eye, and envision your child growing stronger and healthier, bigger and brighter. Take this time to talk to your baby. Speak out loud or convey your intentions through your hands. Most importantly, don't forget to listen back. Your baby may very well have a few things to share with you as well.

Try different hand placements and see what feels best to you. There is no wrong way to do this; it's simply taking the time to connect to that little one within you, taking the time to send your love and to receive your baby's love in return. What a sacred treasure this is to experience! Enjoy every moment of it.

Heart Space to Heart Space

Have you ever heard of the heart space? The heart space is that place within each of us that radiates with the light of our truest, most genuine, most enlightened and evolved self, the space that sings our current truth and dances to the tune of our highest potential. This exercise will connect your own heart space to your baby's heart space so you can begin to get to know each other on a deeper and more intimate level.

Sit comfortably, crisscrossing the legs in the easy position (one leg in front of the other, not on top) or bending the knees and opening your legs up to help your middle section expand. Place one hand on your chest and one hand on your sweet belly. Close your eyes, breathing slow, easy, full breaths. Go deep within and connect to your highest, most loving energy, your heart space. Feel that love swirling and glowing within you. Think now about your baby; see your child as a loving, thinking, individual human being. You might visualize a ray of light connecting your own heart space to your baby's heart space, bonding you heart to heart and soul to soul. Use this connection to convey to your baby your intention to create a loving, safe environment for them. Let your baby feel the love from your heart flow into his or hers. Take some time to imagine what your baby might want you to know. Who is your child? What does your baby want and need from you? What does your child feel for you already, and what does your child feel from you? What will your baby want to do in this life, and how can you help them pursue these passions? Breathe deeply, slowly, and fully into this space of loving exchange between heart spaces.

Connecting to the Earth with Baby

Place your hands on your belly and feel the energy of your own heartbeat. Think of your baby's heart beating within you, and imagine your pulses coming into alignment to produce one perfect pounding beat. Now think of the ground beneath you, the earth below your feet. Can you feel the earth's heart beating as well? Imagine that powerful energy flowing up from the earth, through your body, and into your baby's body. How does your baby respond to this earth energy? Pay heed to any messages, emotions, or visions that come to you. This exercise will help your baby get ready for birth while giving you a chance to get to know your child a little better in the meantime.

More Ways to Send Messages to Baby

Here are some other quick and easy ways to communicate with your baby-to-be throughout the day:

- *Belly Drum.* Simply by drumming your belly gently with your hands and speaking words that match the drumbeats, sounds will easily and rhythmically transfer into your baby. Pat your belly with both hands simultaneously while focusing on and uttering a single word or sound such as the holy syllable "Om." You can also try assigning a different word or sound to each hand. For example, you might pat with your right hand and say the word "love," then pat with your left hand as you say the word "light." Choose your own words and sounds, and keep their meanings clearly in mind. Think about the energies and messages you want to convey to your baby as you drum on your belly.

- *Speak to Your Belly.* Talk to your baby as often as you can. You might talk about what you're doing throughout the day, how excited you are to be a mom, or how much fun your child will have exploring the world. Studies show that babies may begin learning language as early as ten weeks before birth, so chat freely to your belly and don't bother feeling self-conscious about it. You are giving your baby an advantage. Deep bass voices may be the easiest for your baby to pick up through the womb, so you might want to lower your natural speaking voice an octave every now and then. Be sure to invite your partner and any other special people in your life to talk to your belly, too.

- *Sing.* Singing or chanting creates a rhythmic flow of energy throughout your body that your baby is likely to feel and enjoy. You can sing classic nursery songs, popular songs, or songs of your own composition. You might chant an ancient Hindu mantra or create a special chant just for you and your baby.

- *Play Music.* If you're not much of a singer and chanting isn't your thing, try playing ready-made music for your baby. You can play classical music, tribal drumming, healing music, funk, rap, jazz— anything you feel your baby might enjoy or find interesting. You can even buy a special belt to wear around your belly that has a holster for an iPod or other music player and built-in speakers that point inward to send the music right to the baby.

- *Touch That Belly.* Place your hands on your tummy regularly and send the baby your feelings of love and happiness through your touch. Allow others to touch your belly too, if you feel comfortable. It's very unlikely that a person would touch a pregnant belly with ill intentions, so why not let the people you trust touch your growing belly and send to the baby their own positive energies and well wishes? You have every right to set your personal space boundaries exactly where you want them, of course, and those boundaries should be respected. If you don't want a particular person to touch your belly, tell them so. The baby feels everything through you, so if you don't feel comfortable, the baby isn't likely to feel comfortable either.

- *Stop and Notice.* Pay attention to how your baby responds to different stimuli and situations. Does your baby move toward your hand when you touch your belly? Does the baby wiggle around or kick more when there is music playing? How does your baby respond to different voices? Let the baby show you who they are.

Journaling to Baby

Journaling to your baby is another way you can begin embracing and empowering your inner mama right now, before you give birth. By writing about your feelings, hopes, dreams, and fears, you will learn a lot about yourself that you can share with your child later on when the time is right. Through journaling, you can clearly and precisely set your intentions for your pregnancy and have an easier time staying in alignment with those goals.

If you decide to keep a pregnancy journal, choose an attractive hardcover journal or notebook that appeals to you. You can use something ordinary, but a sturdier journal will likely last longer and attract your attention more often. Include in your journal anything you like, from notes about doctor appointments and ultrasound photos to random thoughts and daydreams that come to you throughout the day. Let the journal be an opportunity to share with your children who you are as a person, before you became their mother. Write about your hopes and dreams, as well as the hopes and dreams you have for your child. Set your intentions for both pregnancy and motherhood; write down your goals and the main things you want to accomplish or experience at each stage of the journey. Express through the journal your excitement about welcoming this brand-new little spirit into the world.

You might organize the journal into sections, designating certain pages for keeping track of physical changes and new developments, certain pages for writing about your thoughts and feelings, certain pages for noting odd pregnancy dreams, certain pages for tracking spiritual and magickal experiences during pregnancy, or whatever other sections you deem desirable. You might create headings and subheadings for different topics in the journal, or you can simply write each entry as a personalized letter to your child. You might even sign each entry with your new name: Mom.

Here is an example of what such a journal entry might look like. This one happens to be the first entry from the journal kept by one of your authors here, Emily:

Dear Baby,

This is my first letter to you ... whoever you may be. We found out today that you had chosen us for your parents, and we took a pregnancy test ... or three ... to find out for sure that you are indeed inside me! They say you are only the size of a poppy seed right now ... I can't imagine!

Yesterday, we did a sweat lodge and I prayed for you. Today, I found out you are here. I would not have done the whole sweat if I had taken the test yesterday instead of today. I'm hoping this only results in the strengthening of your faith, and not any damage from the heat.

I am not exactly sure when you were conceived, but I think it was this past week while we were out of town. So far, people seem to think that is too soon for a pregnancy test to be able to detect it. But for me, my body felt it this week. I took yoga every day while I was there, and held my hands on my belly and prayed for you to come—and you answered!

My prayers today are this:

May you be incredibly healthy, strong, and passionate.

I pray that we nourish your spirit, your creativity, and your calling on this earth.

I know that you chose us for a reason. I would love to support you in that reason.

I pray that your dad and I both live very long, strong, healthy lives and that you do also.

I want to watch you grow up into the person you are going to become. I want to be here to see all of it. I am so excited for you to be in our lives! I welcome you with open arms and a loving heart.

Love,

Mom

Journaling offers you an opportunity to explore your feelings about motherhood and cultivate a positive and hopeful outlook. It also gives you a chance to introduce yourself to your child from the space you are currently in, before your baby gets here. It's harder than you might think to recount who you were in your pre-baby days, once that baby arrives and changes the game forever. This is a time of blessings and light. Cherish each and every moment of it and chronicle that excitement so you can one day share it with your child.

Chapter 5

~~~ ୬·୯ ~~~

Pregnancy Dreams Deciphered

Dreams can be mystifying, magickal, and odd at any stage of life, but during pregnancy, dreams can go beyond ordinary weirdness into the realm of the utterly bizarre. Women around the world report more vivid, intense, and strange dreams during pregnancy. It makes sense; not only are your emotions and hormones in high gear, but you're also more likely to sleep more often and wake up during the night more often, which leads to an increase in dreaming and a greater chance of remembering those dreams. We also naturally have more fears and doubts to deal with when we're pregnant, more going on in our subconscious and conscious minds alike. Dreams provide an outlet for expressing and exploring our thoughts and emotions, which are often especially confusing, conflicting, and intense during pregnancy.

Your dreams are bound to get pretty wild during this time, so try not to be too alarmed by any particular dream. At the same time, however, by giving us a glimpse of the subconscious, our dreams can offer us insights and valuable tidbits of information that might not have come to our attention otherwise. Dreams also offer a medium through which spirits and other entities might communicate important messages. Many people have experienced dreams of a deceased loved one appearing with some final gem of wisdom or encouragement to share, while many pregnant women report dreams in which they receive the name of their future child as if through divine inspiration.

Dreaming is a powerful tool we can use to overcome fears, gain psychic insight, divine the future, and more. In this chapter, you'll glean some tips and suggestions for unlocking the secrets of your dreams and harnessing their unique power.

Making the Most of Dreams

By making regular attempts to notice and decipher your dreams, you send a message to the universe that you are ready to make the most of your time spent dreaming. Your dreams will then become more profound and more productive, helping you to better process daily experiences and life-altering transformations.

There are a few things to keep in mind to utilize your dreamtime to the fullest. For starters, make sure you're getting adequate rest so you will actually have a chance to dream. Dreaming is important, so make time for it. Also remember to respect your dreams. Pay attention to the messages you receive in dreams that seem prophetic, and do your best to heed any relevant warnings and act on any useful information that comes to you. Lastly, keep in mind that the ways in which you might utilize your dreams are limited only by your imagination and intentions. You might use your dreamtime to learn the future, overcome obstacles, attract resources, or any other goal. Just practice regularly, set your intentions before you drift off to sleep, and follow the additional tips in this chapter.

Prophetic Dreams vs. Everyday Dreams

Dreams help us to process the confusing flood of information and emotion that flows through our brains every day. Memories are consolidated, information is classified, and emotions are processed. Our dreams often mesh fantasy situations with real-life memories, fears, and desires, leading to some strange scenarios in the dreamworld. So many dreams seem to be pure nonsense, and yet we've all had those occasional dreams that seem like something more, like a prophetic vision of the future or a warning of what's to come. While our bodies sleep, our spirits are free to travel the astral plane, and on this plane we can receive relevant and beneficial messages. Many of these messages come to us in the form of symbols: an enemy shows up as a snake or a real-life obstacle appears as a raging river. You don't want to miss such messages, but at the same time you don't want to live in fear with the expectation that a giant pizza will soon be chasing you down just because you dreamed about it.

It's important to learn how to distinguish between everyday dreams and prophetic dreams. Use the following checklist to help you determine if your dream is prophetic or ordinary, everyday dream nonsense:

- Did something happen in your waking life that could explain the dream? For instance, did you watch a monster movie and then dream about a monster? Dream symbols anchored to real-life experiences are less likely to be prophetic than symbols that appear seemingly out of the blue.

- Do you have anything going on physically that could explain the dream? Real-life pain and discomfort often transfer to our experiences in the dream world. If you're wearing tight-fitting pajamas and you dream of being trapped and confined, there's likely a connection. Likewise, if you have aching legs and you dream you've injured yourself in a race, the dream is probably linked to the real-life pain. On the other hand, dreaming of pain that doesn't have a real-world link can be a cause for attention.

- Have you had the dream more than once? Recurring dreams are more likely to have important messages for us. Write down such dreams so that hopefully you can get a fuller picture of any messages contained therein.

- Is the dream vivid? We're more likely to remember the details of prophetic dreams than of everyday dreams.

- Are you aware in the dream of the fact that you are dreaming? Lucid dreaming can be a signal that important messages and prophecies may be coming through to you while you sleep.

- Do any particular symbols or occurrences that happened in the dream stand out to you? Elements of your dreams that demand attention, aspects you're reminded of well after you wake, often deserve further exploration. Make a note of any such symbols so that you can study them further and have a record of the event in case you dream something similar again.

- Is the dream a serial dream? Sometimes important information is revealed to us in our dreams over a period of time, as if each individual dream is an installment, or episode, of the whole story. Pay attention to dreams that happen in installments, as they are likely to contain relevant messages for you.

Remembering Your Dreams

In order to interpret your dreams, you have to first remember them. There are a few easy things you can do to improve your ability to recall your dreams. One effective technique is to set your intentions before you fall asleep. As you lie in bed, relax your body and let your thoughts flow freely for a few minutes. Then think about the kind of dreams you'd like to have. Would you like your dreams to provide you with some extra insight or guidance on a particular matter? Would you like to utilize your dreams to help you discover how to overcome obstacles in your waking life? Do you just want to get a peaceful night's rest full of pleasant, soothing dreams?

Whatever it is you're looking for in your dreamtime, set your mind to it. Tell yourself you will have the particular types of dreams you want, and tell yourself that you will remember those dreams when you wake. Some people find it helpful to write down these intentions on a piece of paper that's then tucked beneath the pillow or slipped inside the pillowcase. You might also try putting a sprinkling of fresh rose petals beneath your pillow, as this is a charm reputed to improve dream recall.

Another thing you can do to improve your dream recall is to start a dream journal. Keep a notebook and pen beside your bed, and immediately upon waking, write down everything you can remember about your dreams. Even if you don't remember anything, make a note of it. Note the date and time of the dream, and include as many details as you can remember. Go through this routine every single day, and before long, you'll find yourself remembering more and more dreams, and remembering them more vividly as well.

Bad Dreams Aren't Always Bad

Nightmares can cause us to wake up drenched in sweat, submerged in fear, and beset by panic. While occasional nightmares are perfectly normal and perhaps even beneficial, that doesn't make them the least bit more pleasant. Bad dreams can be caused by a variety of factors, including emotional stress or physical stimuli such as pain in a part of the body or an increase in metabolic activity due to a late-night snack. Nightmares might also occur to help us process traumatic events, manage everyday anxieties and fears, and prepare ourselves for possible danger. Some dream experts theorize that dreams could be a biological defense mechanism, simulating potential threats and enhancing the brain's ability to perceive threats and avoid them. We might dream about a threatening scenario as a way to prepare for the situation were it ever to arise, however unlikely that is.

Dream fears, as farfetched and unpleasant as they may be, often represent real fears, and exploring these emotions while we sleep can help us to cope better with these emotions in our waking life. In fact, some research studies have shown that pregnant women who face their fears in the form of nightmares actually have easier labors than pregnant women who don't have nightmares or who don't try to fight back or escape during nightmares.[8]

Even if you're not able to fully overcome your fears while sleeping, just dreaming about these fears and at least attempting to conquer them seems to have a beneficial effect on how we handle real-life fears. The next time you have a nightmare, write it down and see if you can determine the underlying fear that prompted the dream. Explore these emotions objectively, and tell yourself before you fall asleep that your dreams will help you move beyond these fearful feelings.

Deciphering Your Dreams

Modern dream interpretation relies on a mix of psychology, mythology, and traditional and contemporary esoteric or cultural symbolism. When

---

8. Cynthia Dennison Haines, MD, "The Vivid Dreams of Pregnant Women," WebMD, www.webmd.com/baby/features/vivid-dreams-of-pregnant-women.

analyzing your dreams, keep in mind that various symbols may hold an entirely different significance for you than is found in traditional interpretation. Think about what each dream symbol or circumstance means to you in your everyday life, identifying any special connections or unique relationships. For example, to dream of scissors is widely interpreted as being indicative of quarrels and hurtful gossip, but if your everyday waking life has you working as a hairdresser or tailor, then scissors showing up in your dreams could just as likely represent the tools of your chosen trade. Likewise, if you keep dreaming about a robin and your own name happens to be Robin, then you might interpret the bird in your dreams as a symbol of yourself, in addition to or instead of attributing to it its traditional meaning of renewal and new starts.

While dream guides like the one presented here can be helpful in providing clues to your dream's potential meaning, they don't trump your own personal experience and intuition. Keep notes of any dream symbols that seem significant, write down your first impressions, consult a dream guide, and look back over your notes in a few weeks or so to see if any of the symbols become more clear or to determine if there are any patterns developing. Doing so will help you gain clues and insights that will help you understand your dreams on a deeper level.

Pregnancy Dream Symbols Unraveled

Here is a sampling of symbols that often appear in the dreams of pregnant women. This is by no means a definitive guide to dream interpretation. Consult a general dream dictionary for help with any symbols not included here, as we've listed only the ones that most commonly occur during pregnancy.

Angel: To dream of angels can signify spiritual enlightenment, divine blessings, and protection.

Baggage/luggage: Empty luggage signifies a need for greater frugality, while full bags denote a smart budgeting of resources.

Birds: To dream of birds can signify spiritual happiness, freedom, success, and the ability to rise above a challenge or overcome a limitation. To dream of an injured bird can represent fear or sorrow over losses of freedom as the restrictions brought on by pregnancy increase. To dream of a bird in flight denotes gaining control over a situation and can also symbolize expanded awareness, hope, and joy. A flock of birds appearing in a dream can signify prosperity and unexpected surprises. To hear birds singing can prophesy the approach of happy events and celebrations.

Books: To dream of books indicates that you are learning new things and acquiring new knowledge and wisdom.

Bread: To dream of bread symbolizes health, vitality, happiness, good luck, and longevity. If the bread is moldy, burnt, or stale, or if it's being cut or broken, it can signify approaching challenges for which you must prepare.

Bridges: Bridges represent transitions and passages into new stages of life. Dreaming that you're reluctant to cross a bridge reflects hesitation or trepidation about the birthing process and what it will be like to be a mother. Ready or not, your baby is on the way; these dreams are helping you prepare mentally and spiritually for the miracle that's about to happen.

Buildings: Dreaming of architectural structures such as skyscrapers or other buildings mirrors your own growing body and the space inside you where your baby is being formed. Some pregnant women report that these dream buildings get larger and more complete the further along they are. If you feel fearful during such dreams, it could be a reflection of insecurities about your increasing size.

Burying or otherwise hiding something: This dream can indicate that protective feelings are on the rise. It can also symbolize guarding resources or concealing knowledge or opinions.

Butterfly: Dreams of butterflies indicate restlessness followed by a period of great transformation.

Candle: To dream of lighting a candle signifies an approaching birth. A brightly burning candle denotes health, vitality, prosperity, and success, while a faltering flame signifies sadness and delays.

Carrying something: If you dream of carrying packages or other cumbersome items, it may reflect your own feelings of being burdened and overwhelmed in everyday life. Pregnancy is both a blessing and a burden, and these feelings are totally natural. See if you can lessen the stress by letting go of some of your day-to-day obligations. This dream can also be the result of the increased physical pressure you might feel during pregnancy.

Cats: Dreams of cats can signify a happy home life. If the cat is scratching or biting you, however, it can presage strife in intimate relationships.

Chains: To dream of chains indicates repression and restriction and can also symbolize the ill intentions or the contrary, trying nature of people around you.

Coins, money, riches: Money in dreams can signify good luck, a rise in one's station, and new or unrecognized opportunities. To dream of receiving money can symbolize receiving an unexpected blessing. It can also be a symbol of being trusted with something valuable. To dream of giving money can signify letting go of a burden and lessening anxiety. To dream of extreme wealth and opulence can prophesy the birth of a child who will grow up to enjoy a life of prosperity and abundance.

Cows: Dreams of cows presage good luck, fertility, wealth, and prosperity.

Crickets: Good friends and happy times are indicated. The cricket can also be a symbol of wealth and good fortune.

Daffodils: This flower is a symbol of joy and renewal and can presage good news that is on the way.

Daisy: Friendship and true love surround you if you dream of the daisy. It can also be a sign of new friends or good times to come.

Dandelions: Dreams of dandelions can indicate that you are feeling overwhelmed by an influx of other people's ideas and opinions. To dream of these flowers can also be a warning that you are the subject of gossip.

Darkness: Signifying the unknown and/or the repressed, darkness in dreams can take the form of shadowy scenes, darkened rooms, or deep, dark recesses and passages such as underground caves and tunnels. Are there emotions and thoughts you're suppressing, fears with which you have not yet come to terms? Are you disturbed by persistent unanswered questions? Pay attention to your emotional state in these dreams, and don't be afraid to dig deeper once you awaken. By listening to your intuition and/or writing about your dreams, you might be able to discover hidden knowledge you didn't realize you had.

Desert: Feelings of isolation and loneliness; a need for greater spiritual or physical nourishment.

Digging: To dream that you are digging something up signifies good luck, thriftiness, discovering hidden resources, or finding the hidden value in trying situations. To dream of digging a hole signifies that you are digging deep into your subconscious to find what you need right now.

Dock: Safety and protection; escape from potential peril.

Dog: Faithfulness, trustworthy friends, fidelity.

Dolphin: Hope and salvation.

Dropping baby: To dream of dropping, breaking, or otherwise hurting the baby indicates fears about parenting abilities. Know that such dreams are perfectly normal and merely reflect doubts and anxieties that you will need to overcome.

Drowning: To dream you are drowning can indicate emotional exhaustion as you struggle to keep your head above water in waking life. It can also reflect a physical need for more oxygen. Try to improve your posture and take deeper, fuller breaths.

Duck: Good fortune, prosperity, happiness, a child of great beauty.

Eagle: Success and leadership; the birth of a prodigal child who will achieve extraordinary greatness.

Egg: Dreams of eggs are often interpreted as an early sign of pregnancy, representing fertility and the womb. To dream of breaking an egg can signal distress or approaching quarrels, and alternatively can represent the fears that naturally come with pregnancy. If such a dream is recurring frequently or is causing anxiety, you may want to give yourself some extra care and nourishment to help ease your worries.

Elephant: Prosperity, wisdom, fertility.

Erotic dreams: Erotic dreams are common during pregnancy, as our feelings about body image and sexuality are challenged and often transformed during this time. We're less likely to live out our sexual fantasies in waking life, which means these thoughts are more likely to trickle into our dreams.

Fields: If the fields are full of growing things, this dream indicates prosperity and abundance and the culmination of hard work and effort. If the fields are empty and barren, it can indicate disappointment or fears of not having enough to sustain one's self and family.

Fighting/struggling: To dream of fighting indicates that you will gain honor and respect, prevailing over your foes, rivals, and other obstacles.

Fish: Dreams of fish can be an early indicator of pregnancy. Associated with the Chinese goddess Kuan Yin, protector of mothers and children, fish can also symbolize divine protection, good fortune, and blessings. They also signify success to come from endurance and effort.

Flies: Gossip and slander; annoying personalities.

Flowers: Happiness, love, and beauty.

Flying: Greater happiness is on the way.

Fog: Uncertainty, obscured or limited information, having to proceed without full vision of what lies ahead.

Food: To dream of food indicates worry over resources.

Forgetting where you left baby: This dream reflects fears of inadequacy and feeling ill prepared to be a mother. It can also symbolize that you are letting go of something or leaving some aspect of yourself behind as you become a parent.

Forgetting something else: These dreams reflect feelings of being ill prepared for the approaching demands of labor and motherhood.

Do all you can to get ready, then take some deep breaths and try to relax.

Fountain: Health and healing.

Frogs: Dreams of frogs can represent the rapid changes that pregnancy brings. They are also symbols of joy and abundance.

Frost: Difficulties are indicated.

Fruit: Dreams of fruit suggest a time of abundance, hope, enjoyment, and fertility. To dream of eating fruit signifies that you are embracing the blessings of life with full gusto. Rotten or broken fruit can symbolize missed opportunities, often reflecting necessary sacrifices that have been made reluctantly. Specific fruits also carry specific meanings:

> *Apples:* Love, success, peace, and harmony.
>
> *Cherries:* Love and good health.
>
> *Figs:* Prosperity, joy, and pleasure.
>
> *Grapes:* Cheerfulness and prosperity. Stomping grapes indicates the overcoming of obstacles.
>
> *Lemons:* Renewal and new adventures.
>
> *Oranges:* Strength, courage, and energy in spite of anxiety.
>
> *Peaches:* Beauty and passion.
>
> *Pears:* Good luck and prosperity.
>
> *Pomegranates:* Fertility, sensuality, and an abundance of blessings.
>
> *Strawberries:* Happiness and good luck.
>
> *Watermelons:* Happiness, friendship, and the rapid physical growth caused by pregnancy.

Fully grown kid/talking babies: To dream that your baby is born fully grown or already talking indicates excitement, eagerness, and impatience about meeting your new baby and getting to know who your child is. It can also reflect an innate awareness that pregnancy and babyhood are very fleeting, temporary stages that should be cherished and enjoyed while you have the chance.

Gardens: Success, fertility, prosperity, and a swift stroke of good luck.

Giving birth to multiple babies: This dream can signal more babies to come. If you already have several children and dream this dream, it can be a symbol of feeling overwhelmed and doesn't necessarily indicate a future of multiple pregnancies.

Giving birth to other creatures: To dream of giving birth to other creatures is a reflection of the primal instincts that are brought to the forefront during pregnancy. Dreams of giving birth to certain specific animals may also contain particular prophecies regarding your baby's general nature or destiny:

> *Crane:* A long life is indicated.
>
> *Dragon:* A person of power, leadership, and ability.
>
> *Duck:* An extraordinarily beautiful child.
>
> *Elephant:* Wisdom, power, longevity, and prosperity are presaged.
>
> *Elk:* A lucky child.
>
> *Goose:* A silly, playful nature.
>
> *Hawk:* An enterprising and intelligent person; a leader.
>
> *Lamb:* A child who will be valued greatly as a friend.
>
> *Lion:* A person of great courage and strength.
>
> *Monster:* An indication that you need to let go of certain fears and old sorrows. This dream does not reflect on your child's temperament or appearance.
>
> *Mule:* A steadfast, stubborn, reliable nature.
>
> *Nightingale or other songbird:* Great talent in singing or other musical pursuits is indicated.
>
> *Ox:* An obedient, hardworking person.
>
> *Rabbit:* Cleverness, wit, and good luck are indicated.
>
> *Rooster:* A proud nature and a life of power and success.

Hail: Troubles and sorrow.

Hedgehog: A reunion with a friend from the past. Loyalty and honesty.

Hill: To dream of climbing a hill indicates that you are overcoming difficulties. To fail to reach the top can indicate disappointments and a need to rethink your strategy.

Horse: Happiness, courage, success, and generosity are indicated.

Identifying your baby: To dream that you must identify your baby out of a selection of many identical or similar babies is a reflection of the maternal bond developing and deepening.

Iron: Protection and strength.

Leopard: Indicates changes and difficulties that inspire fear or leave you feeling intimidated. Also a symbol of alertness and watchfulness.

Letter: Good news is on the way.

Lilies: Morality and strong ethics will lead to happiness.

Marigolds: Happiness, protection, friendship, and illumination are indicated.

Marsh or swamp: Struggling to overcome difficulties; a slow and perilous passage.

Meadow: Happiness and contentment are presaged.

Mirror: To dream of looking into a mirror can indicate the birth of a child. To dream of breaking a mirror indicates a change in one's self-image or a sudden transformation of identity.

Moon: To dream of the moon indicates divine protection and strong maternal instincts.

Morphed body: Dreaming that your body is morphing into enormous proportions or undergoing other strange transformations is a reflection of your fears and insecurities regarding your changing body.

Names: When you dream about the name of your future child, even if it's a nonsense name, write it down. Such names are said to be magickal and divinely inspired. A name that comes in a dream can be a source of power and protection for your child as they grow, so consider using the name as a nickname or secret name if not the child's actual name.

Nest: A happy home life is indicated.

Ocean: Symbol of life, fertility, and accomplishment. Smooth, clear oceans denote great joy, while dark or turbulent oceans denote sorrow and worry. See also *Water*.

Olives: Indicates happiness, contentment, a rise in station, or an unexpected upturn in fortune.

Packing: Dreams of packing indicate preparations that are being made or that need to be made for baby. To dream of someone helping you pack or carry luggage symbolizes that you have lots of help and support throughout this journey. See also *Baggage/luggage*.

Palm tree: Joy, pregnancy, spiritual happiness.

Pansy: Kindness and faithfulness.

Planting seeds: Presages the establishment of a firm foundation on which a successful and happy future will be created.

Porcupine: A need for diplomacy and delicacy when dealing with troublesome people or situations.

Puddles: There are some undesirable people in your life whose influence you would do best to avoid.

Quicksand: Dreams of quicksand denote temptation, danger, and undiscovered vulnerabilities.

Rabbits: Dreaming about rabbits while pregnant can signify a state of prolific fertility and may be a signal of more children to come.

Raft: Escape from danger.

Rain: Troubles and anxiety. Can also indicate unexpressed sexuality and unfulfilled passions that are overflowing and demanding attention.

Reeds: Decisions must be made.

River: Clear, smoothly flowing water signifies happiness and abundance, while a muddy or turbulent river represents troubles and difficulties. See also *Water*.

Salamander: A dream of reassurance and divine protection.

Searching: To dream that you are searching for something can symbolize that you have left behind a part of yourself or given up on an important goal or dream that you should perhaps reclaim.

Ship: Plans, expectations, the fulfillment of hopes and dreams.

Snakes: To dream of a snake can signal conflicting ideas and personalities, acting as a reminder to trust your own best judgment and not be swayed too much by the opinions of those around you. In China, to dream of a green snake is said to indicate a healthy baby and a happy life, whereas a red snake signals a wedding or an engagement of someone close to you. Dreaming of a black snake is believed to prophesy the birth of a boy, while dreams of a white snake prophesy the birth of a girl. Also a phallic symbol, snakes appearing in dreams can represent sexual needs and desires.

Snow: Difficulties that will be overcome; prosperity.

Sparrow: An unexpected stroke of good luck is headed your way.

Spider: Preparation, perseverance, and foresight. To see a spider spinning a web signals the arrival of money.

Stairs: To dream of going upstairs signifies a rise in station and happiness in love and life, while to dream of going downstairs indicates a descent in position or that you are leaving something behind.

Storms: Temporary misfortunes that will pass.

Swallow: The arrival of news.

Swamp: Money troubles and worries.

Swan: Happiness, wealth, and grace.

Swimming: To dream of swimming with one's head above water signifies success, while struggling to stay afloat signifies obstacles and anxieties that must be overcome.

Trains, railways: Changes and passages.

Turtles: To dream of turtles represents strength, fertility, and protection. Turtles can also symbolize ancestors and other links to the past.

Underground/tunnels/corridors: To dream that you are underground or traveling through a dark tunnel or corridor indicates that you are delving deep into the subconscious mind to tap into strength, energy reserves, and other resources you didn't know you had. If you dream that you successfully make it through such a passage, it can be an indication of anxiety or difficulties that will pass.

Unicorn: Spiritual attainment, intuitive awareness, magickal power and protection.

Visitations by friends, relatives, ancestors: Such dreams may contain direct messages from your loved ones. Write down all you remember. Dreaming of relatives can also be a sign that family ties and bonds of friendship are becoming more important to you now that you have your own family. Examine your feelings about family and set your intention to make your family the best it can be.

Water: From bodies of water such as oceans and rivers to showerheads and kitchen faucets, to dream of water in any form represents emotions. Raging waters signify emotional upheaval or being overwhelmed by emotion, whereas calm or gently flowing water represents emotional joy, contentment, and love. To dream of drinking a glass of clear, fresh water signifies needs being met and emotional satisfaction, while dreaming of drinking dirty water symbolizes discomfort. See also *Ocean* and *River*.

Wind/breezes: A gentle breeze signifies the arrival of happy news, while strong winds presage quarrels between friends and lovers.

Dream a Little Dream

While pregnancy dreams can be bizarre as well as disturbing, they also hold great value. We can gain insight into the future, conquer fears, overcome anxieties, recognize patterns of behavior, and even receive messages from deceased loved ones or from the gods themselves. Don't discount your dreams. What seems like sheer nonsense today could very well make perfect sense tomorrow. Keep a log or dream journal and start writing down everything you remember about your dreams. Read through your notes regularly and jot down any additional insights that may have come to you. Your dreamtime is an essential part of your life, so make the most of it and enjoy it as much as you can.

Chapter 6

~~~~~~~~

Preparing for Birth

As labor nears, it's time to get as ready as possible. While we can never be fully prepared for the challenges and triumphs that will come with delivering a baby into the world, there are many useful techniques you can use and lots of information to explore that will help you feel more confident and ready when it comes time to give birth.

In this chapter, you'll find practical tips, rituals, meditations, and visualizations to help ease your labor and increase the chances of a successful delivery. You'll learn which stones to use to lessen labor pain and speed delivery, and you'll also discover angels, saints, and deities who can be called on by moms for protection, help, and healing for themselves and their babies. The main thing to keep in mind is that each birth experience is unique. Yours will be like no other. By arming yourself with a variety of magickal tools and proven, practical techniques, you'll be better prepared for whatever your own unique birth experience may bring.

Plans, Possibility, and Flexibility

Most pregnancy books include information about different birthing options and which to choose for which reasons. There are many methods to choose from and important decisions to be made, including deciding to have a water birth versus a land birth, a home birth versus a hospital birth, and a natural birth versus having an epidural, and whether to choose a doctor, doula, or midwife. While we recognize these choices as a sacred part of the pregnancy process, we're not going to go into detail about any of these because we know you will be guided to make the decisions that work best for you. You can read all about your many birthing options in other pregnancy books.

What we want to offer here instead is some valuable advice: While it's important to have a birth plan in place, it's equally important to recognize the fact that things will not usually go exactly as you expect. Plan and prepare as you may, there's really no telling what your baby's birth might be like or might require until it's actually happening. You have to become okay with that. It's not about you and your plans when it comes to birth. It's about your baby and bringing your child into the world safely. You may have your heart set on having precisely the kind of birth you dream about and envision, and hopefully it will go just that way. Being overly rigid in your ideas, however, is something you simply cannot afford to do. Plan as much as possible how you want the birth to go, but retain a level of flexibility in those plans. Unexpected circumstances might arise that could throw your carefully thought-out plans right out the window.

If the labor and birth don't go exactly as you imagine and hope, it's important to let go of any guilt or disappointment regarding any unfulfilled expectations. If you dream of a natural birth in a softly lit room with relaxing music playing, for instance, and instead end up having an emergency C-section under the glare of operating-room lights, don't take it too hard. At the end of the day, it's about making the best and safest choices for you and your baby, even if those choices may deviate greatly from the original plan.

That said, it can help you feel more prepared and confident to have a plan in place. Research your options and make the choices that are best, understanding that you may have to alter those plans at the last minute. While you may want to discuss birthing options with other women to gain some personal insight into the different methods, be aware that some people are very opinionated and may try to make you feel guilty or second-guess your choices. If you decide on a home birth, for example, you'll likely hear the argument that you are putting the baby in danger. If you decide on a hospital birth, you'll likely hear the argument that doctors are hack jobs and that millions of women have done it naturally and independently.

Try not to take anyone's judgments or opinions too seriously. This isn't about a storybook birth or what your friends might think of you. This is about your baby, and you should feel confident in your ability to be flexible and make the best choices for your child based on the unique circumstances of your own unique delivery.

Ready for Baby Ritual

This ritual will help you feel better prepared, more optimistic, and more grounded and centered as you anticipate the challenges of labor and the thrill of meeting your new baby. If possible, perform this ritual on the night of the full moon preceding your due date. Choose a space where you can sit comfortably, either in a chair or on the floor with some pillows for support. You will need a small stick covered in bark that can be easily peeled away and removed with the fingers, and a fist-sized lump of modeling clay or children's playdough. Place these items beside you. If you like, put on some soft, relaxing music.

Imagine the space you're in surrounded by an orb of positive, loving energy. You might envision it as a force field of glowing white light. Acknowledge to yourself that you are safe in this space; know that you are surrounded by only good, helpful energies. You might invite into this space any beneficial energies you like, such as angels, deities, nature spirits, or ancestors. Take a few slow, deep breaths to help calm your mind and center your focus.

When you're ready, pick up the stick and think honestly about your fears of giving birth. Allow yourself to dwell on these thoughts for a moment, expressing each fear and addressing each doubt in turn. As you engage in these thoughts, strip away the bark from the outside of the stick, removing it piece by piece. Put the pieces in a pile beside you so you can discard them later. As you peel away each strip of bark, imagine yourself successfully overcoming each fear, each doubt. Know that all you have to do to beat these fears is to face them, and think about how the ritual at hand is preparing you for this future time.

Once you've peeled away all or most of the bark, hold the stick lovingly in your hands as if it were your newborn baby. Imagine yourself holding your own precious child, and let your heart fill with love at this vision. Pick up the lump of clay, and with love in your hands, mold the clay around the stick as you think about how quickly your new baby will grow and develop. Think about your baby's limbs becoming thicker and stronger as you mold the clay; see your child's tiny heart pounding with health and vigor. If you're artistic, mold the clay into the shape of a body. You can even scratch in little eyes, a nose, and a mouth. Hold this little stick baby in your hands and visualize your real baby now in the womb, then being born, and then rapidly turning into a toddler, kid, and adolescent. Think about the fact that labor is just a single step of the adventure; the real journey begins once the baby actually gets here. Know that you will get through the birth of your child successfully. Tell yourself out loud, "I am ready to welcome my child. This is a blessing, and I can do this." If you've called any deities, angels, or other entities to join with you in this ritual, thank them now and ask them to look over you again when the time of delivery approaches.

Now that the ritual is complete, discard the pieces of bark outdoors, covering them with a layer of dirt. Keep the stick with the clay on it in a safe place in your home, perhaps on top of a shelf or dresser or in an open box that you can use like a miniature cradle. Just don't cram it in a drawer somewhere and forget about it; you want to leave it out in the open so you can look at it often and remind yourself that you are ready to welcome your child. If you like, surround the stick baby each day with offerings of flowers, fruit, coins, milk, or other trinkets as you express your gratitude, confidence, and love for your blessing to come.

Goddesses, Angels, and Saints for Healing, Help, and Protection

Sometimes we need a little extra support during pregnancy and labor, support that reaches well beyond the physical to touch our very soul. Whether your worldview includes gods, goddesses, angels, saints, or other divine entities, there is much help to be had from the realm of Spirit. Little of that help will come if it isn't solicited, so ask. Connect to whatever entities or spirits you believe in, and ask for their help, love, strength, and guidance.

You may choose to work with one of the mother goddesses discussed in Chapter 4: Embracing Your Inner Mama. You may choose to work with a patron saint, deity, or spirit guide. We each connect to different aspects of the divine in unique ways, and the particular entities you personally acknowledge and work with are completely a matter of personal choice. If you need some inspiration, however, here is a sampling of goddesses, angels, and saints that many mothers have turned to for healing, help, or protection during pregnancy and labor. If any appeal to you, consider investigating them further and possibly employing their aid during this special time.

Archangel Gabriel: This angel is revered for his ability to render help to both mother and child from conception till birth and beyond.

Archangel Metatron: This angel helps protect babies during childbirth and beyond and is known for his special fondness for indigo children, crystal children, starseed children, and lightworkers.

Archangel Michael: Archangel Michael is known as a great protector. Call on this brave archangel to keep you and your baby safe in times of danger or difficulty.

Archangel Raphael: This angel is also known as the "medicine of God." If you or your baby are in need of healing, this is the angel to call on.

Carmenta: This Roman goddess of childbirth and prophecy can be called upon for an easy and swift delivery. She is traditionally presented with offerings of rice.

Deverra: This Roman goddess can be called upon to watch over the mother's safety during labor. Her symbol is a broom, which has the power to sweep away evil energies.

Frigg: This Nordic goddess can be petitioned to help ease labor pains and speed the delivery. Wife to the god Odin, she is also associated with the earth and the atmosphere.

Ishtar: This Babylonian mother goddess can be called on to help guard the mother's health during pregnancy. She can also be petitioned for protection of the baby during childbirth and beyond.

Isis: This Egyptian goddess is a fierce protector of mothers and their children. She is the daughter of Geb the earth god and Nut the sky goddess. Patroness of nature and magick, Isis is particularly helpful to the downtrodden and others in need.

Ixchel: Associated with the moon and with water, this Mayan goddess also presides over pregnancy and labor. Her symbol is a jug filled with water.

Kuan Yin: This Buddhist and Taoist goddess is also known as the Blessed Mother. A very comforting energy to call near, she will help heal, nourish, and protect both you and your baby.

Mother Mary: This Roman Catholic conception of the divine mother can be called on for help and protection during pregnancy and labor. Also known as the Blessed Virgin Mother, she is often petitioned to help ease pain and bring comfort when we're in the midst of life's especially trying moments.

Ngolimento: This Ewe goddess watches over the baby and protects the child's soul throughout the pregnancy. She is the mother of spirits.

Nona: Her name meaning "nine," this Roman goddess is called on for protection particularly during the ninth months of pregnancy. Nona belongs to a triad of goddesses called the Parcae, who were the rulers of destiny in ancient Roman mythology.

Periyachi: This goddess of Hindu origin is known in Singapore as well as Malaysia. She is a fierce protector of babies and children and will help guard the child during pregnancy and birth.

Saint Anthony: This Catholic saint is known as the patron saint of children. He can be petitioned for help whenever you need special protection for your baby.

Saint Gerard: The patron saint of mothers during pregnancy and conception, Saint Gerard is venerated in Catholicism for his protective and nurturing qualities, which are reputed to shield expectant mothers from pain as well as danger.

Tamayorihime: This Japanese sea goddess presides over the embryonic fluids to help keep both mother and baby safe throughout the birth. She can also be petitioned to guard fertility, increase good luck, and avert disaster.

Visualizations for an Easier Labor

Giving birth can be a frightening prospect. Visualization is a powerful tool that can help you reduce anxiety and manage the pains of labor. Our experiences are heavily tinted by our own unique perceptions and expectations. If we think our labor pains will be just awful, they likely will be, while if we instead imagine we will be able to successfully manage the birth process, those real-life pains-to-come will affect us far less. Visualization can be used well before labor to prepare the mind, body, and spirit to face the experience of childbirth with courage and confidence, and it can also be employed for pain relief and anxiety reduction during labor and delivery. Try the following ideas or create your own personal imagery that speaks to you.

Visualization to Prepare the Mind, Body, and Spirit for Childbirth

When we visualize success, we're more likely to achieve it. By envisioning your labor process as successful, you can help minimize fear and anxiety and better prepare yourself for this momentous occasion. Well before your due date, take some time to visualize yourself having the baby. Imagine yourself enduring each stage of labor with courage, determination, and stamina. Visualize the labor progressing quickly and easily. Envision yourself feeling confident and able, inside and out, and mentally and spiritually prepared.

As you imagine the later stages of the delivery, visualize your body as strong, resilient, and flexible. If you are having a vaginal delivery, imagine yourself pushing the baby down and out of the birth canal easily. See the baby moving swiftly and safely out of your womb and into the waiting arms of the world. If you are having a C-section birth, imagine your baby being lifted out of your womb to greet the surrounding environment.

Visualize your baby taking his or her first breaths outside of your body; imagine your child's first cries. See yourself smiling, holding your healthy newborn lovingly in your arms. Repeat this visualization often as your time of labor nears.

Visualizations for Pain Management During Labor

By creating alternative visual imagery to shift your focus away from the pain your body is experiencing, you can change your perception of that pain and greatly reduce your discomfort. Choose an image well ahead of time so you'll be prepared when the first waves of labor pain strike. You might imagine that each painful sensation is a rocket shooting you higher and higher into the sky toward the glowing stars for which you're aiming. You might visualize your cervix expanding and your baby descending further down the birth canal with each throbbing pang of pressure and discomfort. You might envision your vagina as a lotus, its center opening wider and wider as each wave of pain comes and goes.

If such imagery is a bit too fluffy and flowery for your taste, envision something different. You might visualize yourself throwing a rock through a pane of glass, shattering it into a million pieces with each crashing pain. You might imagine your fist smashing into a brick wall, breaking it down easily as you pound through your discomfort. You might imagine yourself as a fierce eagle, piercing through a stormy sky as you rise above your physical sensations.

Some women find it helpful to visualize a field of solid color. You might choose a healing shade such as white, lavender, or emerald green. As each pain hits, envision the color enveloping your whole body in a glowing orb, infusing you with strength, diminishing discomfort, and bringing a sense of peace and contentment.

Pre-Labor Meditation for Mothers-to-Be

Meditation is another technique you can employ well before labor hits to get yourself as centered and ready as possible. Meditation triggers the body to go into relaxation mode. Muscle tension is released and the body's systems function more efficiently. The areas of the brain governing consciousness, memory, learning, and the perception of happiness become more active. Stress and pain are diminished and a sense of calm and joy fill the heart. During meditation, our everyday thoughts and fears take a back seat as we focus instead on the act of meditation. With regular practice, we learn to retain that sense of meditative calm in our day-to-day happenings and doings, helping us to cope better with daily stress and handle bigger challenges such as the prospect of giving birth.

Find a quiet place where you can sit or lie down comfortably without interruption. You don't need a whole lot of time, but the more you have, the better. However, in a pinch, a good five to fifteen minutes of meditation will do wonders. The key to meditation is to silence the conscious mind while listening to the subconscious mind. Repetition is one way to achieve this state. You might focus on the repetition of your breath, paying attention to each inhalation and exhalation, limiting your mental activity to this single point of interest. You might play a CD of a simple drumbeat, letting the cyclical rhythm fill your mind and body completely. You might observe the back and forth motion of a swinging clock chime, a metronome, or the swaying leaves on a windswept tree. The point of focus doesn't matter as much as the fact that you are shifting your attention away from your everyday thoughts and onto something you find relaxing.

Try to get as zoned out as possible while meditating; put your doubts and anxieties on hold for a moment. Don't try too hard but rather go with the flow, letting your thoughts come and go and paying them as little heed as possible. Striving has no place in meditation; the only goal is to relax. Try to practice meditation regularly, as its benefits are cumulative. As your time of labor nears, do your best to meditate daily, even if only for a few minutes. If you do, you'll have a good chance of a less painful and less stressful labor.

Meditating During Labor

Meditation is also useful during childbirth. While trying to completely empty your mind when it's filled with pain and distress is next to impossible, you can still benefit from incorporating adapted meditation techniques into the birthing process. Try distracting yourself from physical discomfort and mental stress by focusing on a mantra, a type of sacred chant used in meditative practices to align and harmonize the spirit. You can use a traditional mantra such as the holy syllable "Om," which symbolizes the totality of the divine made manifest, or you can create your own personal mantra that speaks specifically to your own experience. For instance, when a labor pain overwhelms you, you might repeat in your head the chant "good mama, strong mama" or something even simpler like "I'm okay" or "I can, I will." The repetition will provide a measure of distraction and relief from the stresses of labor.

It can also be helpful to incorporate mudras, or sacred hand shapes, into your labor meditation. Mudras are believed to help align and activate various energy circuits that course through the body. During the delivery, try utilizing the *prithvi mudra*. With your palm facing outward, touch the tip of your ring finger to the tip of your thumb and extend the other fingers upward. This hand position is used to center and stabilize your energies, increase patience, and boost endurance to help you get through the delivery as smoothly and calmly as possible.

If this mudra feels odd or uncomfortable to you, try a different hand movement. You might make little circles with your wrists, your fingers together and extended. You might simply alternate between making a tight fist and loosening it, letting your fingers spread wide and stretch out as far as possible. Whatever movement or mantra you choose, the repetition of such techniques can be beneficial in relaxing and shifting your focus to help you cope more confidently with the pain of having a baby.

Another hand shape you might try is the *vishnu mudra*. Bring together your thumb and index finger. It's believed that the thumb represents the universe and the index finger represents you. Doing this hand position connects you to the universe, centering and balancing your energies. Breathe slowly and deeply, concentrating on the flow of energy within your hands. This hand position will help you to regain a sense of calm and control. Just do the hand gesture and then look to see what the moment brings.

Magickal Childbirth Sachet

A magickal sachet is essentially a bundle of herbs and other ingredients that have been wrapped up in cloth, bound with string, and infused with prayers, wishes, and other intentions. You can make your own special sachet to use as a protective charm to help bring good fortune to both you and your baby throughout your pregnancy and during the birth. Start by choosing a small square of cloth in a color attuned to your particular prayer or aim. For instance, you might select baby blue, pink, or pale yellow to represent the baby, green for healing, or white for purity and protection. Next, choose a mixture of herbs to help represent your wishes and convey them to the powers that be. You might use sage to symbolize protection, purity, and wisdom. You might choose rosemary to represent love and success. You might choose cinnamon to bring extra strength and courage, or you might select basil to represent good luck and fine health.

Whatever herb you choose, mix it with a pinch of sage and/or a pinch of cornmeal. Infused with nurturing, stabilizing energies, the cornmeal will help ground your intentions, aligning and connecting your will to the strength of Mother Earth, while the sage will act as a doorway to the spirit realm, carrying your wishes up to the heavens. Place the mixture on the center of the cloth. Mix it up a little more as you think of your particular wishes coming true. Visualize the successful pregnancy and birth you want to have, and put the energy of these thoughts into the herbs. Imagine a glowing energy flowing out of your fingertips and into the mix as you touch it. Do this slowly, intently, and with a full heart; don't rush it. Twist the cloth into a little bundle, and tie it at the top to secure the contents. If you plan to wear your magickal childbirth sachet as a necklace, use a long piece of string to tie it at the top so the loose ends will be large enough to fit comfortably around your neck.

Once it's all tied up, hold the finished sachet in your hands and think clearly of your goal once more as you breathe these intentions into the little bundle. You can make several childbirth sachets if you like, each representing a different prayer or wish. You may want to invite your loved ones to make a special sachet for you as well.

Keep your magickal childbirth sachets close to your body to help bring a little extra luck as your due date nears. You may want to carry them with you into the birthing room so you can hold them in your hands for extra comfort and reassurance. As an alternative, you might burn the sachets prior to the birth, envisioning the smoke carrying your desires into the spirit realm. Some people like to wait until after the birth to burn the sachets, using the ceremony as a way to express gratitude and mark the end of this sacred, life-changing, life-giving experience. Of course, you may want to save a childbirth sachet to keep as a special memento and souvenir from your pregnancy. Magickal sachets can be formed for any purpose and can be used in many ways. If and how you choose to employ them during pregnancy and labor depends entirely on your own needs, desires, and inspiration.

Tsue Shen Ritual for a Speedy Delivery

In Chinese culture, a timely, safe, and swift delivery is encouraged through a tradition called *tsue shen*, which translates as "hastening delivery." Roughly one month before the baby is due, the expectant mother's mother will send to her a package of new clothes for herself and a special gift for the baby—a white cloth or blanket that is to be wrapped around the baby once the child is born.[9] This simple gesture symbolizes the continuity of family and encourages the baby to arrive on time. If the tsue shen ritual inspires you, you might ask your mother or another maternal woman in your life to mail to you a package a month before your due date. The white cloth or blanket is the essential element; any other mama clothes, baby clothes, or other trinkets are icing on the cake. Bring this special blanket with you to the delivery, and wrap it around your newborn child as soon as is reasonable.

Knot Magick for Mothers

In Transylvania, Finland, Scotland, the East Indies, West Africa, North America, and other places around the world, women have employed

---

9. Shu Shu Costa, *Lotus Seeds and Lucky Stars: Asian Myths and Traditions About Pregnancy and Birthing* (New York: Simon & Schuster, 1998), 43.

the ancient art of knot magick to ease the pains and difficulties of child-birth.[10] Knots in clothing are undone and braided hair is let loose in an act of sympathetic magick intended to "loosen" the womb and clear away any obstacles that might otherwise delay or hinder the delivery.

To try your own bit of knot magick, you might consider creating a special knotted cord prior to the delivery so you can undo this knot for a powerful burst of magick when the time of labor nears. Choose a red, white, or green cord to represent the womb. Tie a single knot in the middle of the cord while envisioning your baby remaining safe and sound inside your womb until the day of birth arrives. As you tie the knot, say, "I tie this knot; I tie it tight. Stay inside till the time is right!" When labor approaches, undo the knot as you say, "I untie the knot; I open the way. Safe and soon will I meet my baby today!"

Birth Beads

Birth beads are a string of beads that can be worn or held for extra energy, luck, or protection during pregnancy and childbirth. Birth beads contain the energies of all those who have previously used them, so they often become treasured family heirlooms, passed down through the family and used by generation after generation.

If you don't have a set of birth beads already, consider starting a new family tradition by creating your own special strand infused with all the magick and intention you desire. Wooden beads, crystal beads, glass beads, or stone beads are all great choices due to their durability and positive energy. You may even consider creating your own beads, forming each bead out of clay that can be hardened in the oven or painting ready-made beads by hand to give them your own personal touch.

The number of beads you include in your strand of birth beads is up to you. Each bead can be linked to a different desire, prayer, energy, or intention. For example, one bead might represent endurance, another may represent luck, and yet another might hold a special wish for an easy labor or for a beautiful, healthy child. Choose a sturdy string or ribbon on which

10. Sir James George Frazer, *The Golden Bough* (1922), Chapter 21, Section 11, "Knots and Rings Tabooed," www.bartleby.com/196/54.html.

to place the beads, and tie a large knot or loop at the end to keep the beads from sliding off as you work. Affirm your intentions as you string each bead.

Keep the birth beads close to you, and handle them whenever you feel you need a little extra comfort, energy, or encouragement. They can be very beneficial during the delivery, providing you with another avenue of focus when the pains of labor become overwhelming. Hold on tight to the birth beads while pushing. Squeeze them as hard as you like—they won't break. Let the energy of the beads flow into you and strengthen you, and put the energy of all the bliss and pain of your own unique pregnancy and birth back into the beads.

Cut the Pain Charm

Among rural folk in the Ozarks, one curious custom was to place a knife under the mattress of the pregnant woman during labor. This was believed to cut the pain of the delivery in half.[11] A similar custom is practiced in China but for a different reason. In Chinese culture, a knife placed under the bed of a pregnant woman is believed to frighten away any evil spirits that might otherwise seek to harm the child.[12]

You might have to get a little creative if you'd like to try some knife magick at your delivery, especially if you've chosen a traditional hospital setting. It might be impossible to use a real metal knife, but there are several simple yet effective substitutions you can employ. A plastic knife, a thorn, a needle, a sharp twig, a small pair of manicure scissors, or even a nail file can be used to the same effect. Simply place the object beneath the mattress or under the bed. If this is impossible, try to keep it close by in a handbag, pocket, or drawer. You might designate a friend who will be with you during labor to have the knife or knife-substitute on their person throughout the delivery.

---

11. Janet L. Allured, "Women's Healing Art: Domestic Medicine in the Turn-of-the-Century Ozarks," Bernard Becker Medical Library Digital Collection, http://beckerexhibits.wustl.edu/mowihsp/articles/Ozarks.htm.

12. Debbie Bird, "Pregnancy Customs," BabyWorld, October 1, 2011, http://posts.mode.com/pregnancy-customs.

Top Ten Stones for Pregnancy and Childbirth

Various rocks have been used by pregnant women in many cultures around the world to help promote a healthy and easy delivery. These rocks may be held in the hand, kept near the place of birth, or incorporated into jewelry to be worn throughout pregnancy or specifically at the time of labor. Consider utilizing any of the following stones for extra comfort and support as you get ready to welcome your baby.

Aetite: Reduces the pain of labor and helps prevent premature birth.

Bloodstone: Reduces pain, promotes healing, increases circulation, and protects both mother and baby.

Clear Quartz: Eases pain, magnifies strength and confidence, and helps ensure a successful pregnancy and delivery.

Emerald: Reduces the pain and difficulties of delivery and protects the mother throughout the pregnancy and birth.

Malachite: Speeds delivery, eases pain, protects the baby during birth, and encourages a positive outlook.

Moonstone: Relaxes the nerves, reduces fear, protects the mother during labor, and aids in lactation.

Moss Agate: Reduces pain, eases labor, protects against complications, and increases confidence.

Onyx: Increases stamina, reduces pain, protects the mother, and speeds delivery.

Rose Quartz: Relieves stress, aligns the energies of mother and baby, and soothes pain during and after childbirth.

Ruby: Helps promote a healthy pregnancy and safe delivery.

Childbirth Charm Bag

For an extra helping of good luck and magickal protection during your delivery, try creating this childbirth charm bag. Begin by choosing two or more of the stones just mentioned. Hold the stones in your hand as you think of their magickal properties. Feel the energy of the stones pulsating, and envision this vibration growing in strength so that it surrounds your whole body in a field of soothing, protective power. Imagine yourself experiencing a safe, easy delivery free of complications. Next, cut out a small circle of green or white fabric and place the stones in the middle. Gather the fabric and tie at the top with a white thread, just like you would do if you were making an herbal sachet. For extra potency, anoint the stones or the cloth with lavender, frankincense, neroli, or rose essential oil. Carry this charm bag with you in the delivery room, and squeeze it when you need a little extra luck or support.

Ready or Not

The tips and tools you learned in this chapter can boost your confidence, increase your readiness, and help your delivery go much smoother. Just keep in mind that however many preparations you make and plans you devise, you'll never be totally 100 percent ready and prepared for childbirth, and you can never be 100 percent certain what to expect. Even if you've had other children, each birth experience is bound to be unique, filled with its own unusual elements and humorous occurrences that will all blend to create a wonderful story that you will tell again and again. Just like you and your baby, your pregnancy story will be one of a kind. Embrace yours in whatever form it unfolds.

Chapter 7

~~~ ᦞᦞ ~~~

Welcoming Baby

The challenges of pregnancy have ended while the challenges of motherhood have just begun. This is a time to both take a deep breath and let out a big sigh as you brace yourself for the realities of taking care of a baby 24/7. It can be a demanding task, to say the least, but the joys of seeing your little baby grow and develop, smile and laugh and coo, far outweigh the frustrations that must be endured along the way. In this chapter, you'll find some ideas for celebrating your new baby and sailing smoothly through the first challenges that motherhood may bring.

Baby Blessing Rituals Around the World

People around the world welcome their newborn babies with a variety of rituals and traditions. From christenings and Wiccanings to a simple exchange of gifts or a family feast, the ways in which we welcome our babies vary according to culture, time, and personal taste. Read on to discover some interesting baby-blessing rituals from around the world, then create your own special rituals and traditions that suit you best.

Thailand Book and Pencil Custom

In Thailand, a special custom is practiced on the first three nights of a newborn baby's life. Traditionally, the baby was to spend the first few nights in a special bed called a *kradong*, a type of woven basket-tray with low sides into which bedding was placed. Beneath the kradong, various items were stowed in order to ensure the child would acquire the skills necessary for success in life. In older times, a knife and sickle were placed under the kradong so the child would grow up to acquire skills in agriculture and warfare. Today, actual kradongs are uncommon and parents may opt to place items beneath the ordinary baby crib or cradle. The items have also changed. Instead of a knife and sickle, many modern parents place a book and a pencil, symbols of the good education necessary for success in today's world. Sometimes money is placed beneath the bed to help ensure a life free from material want.[13]

You might be inspired to create your own similar yet unique tradition. For instance, you might place a heart-shaped pendant or a rose petal beneath your baby's bed to ensure a life filled with love, or put a small statue of a bluebird under the bed to symbolize a happy life. As long as the symbolism makes sense to you, the charm will be effective.

Ainu Custom for Protection Against Disease and Illness

Unlike many modern people who prefer brand-new clothing for their infants, the Ainu, an indigenous people of Japan, preferred to dress their babies in clothes made from old, well-worn fabric. The older, less desirable fabric was believed to repel demons of disease and illness that might otherwise sicken or injure the baby out of envy.[14] On a more practical, mundane level, older fabric is soft to the touch and feels more comfortable against the baby's delicate skin.

This ancient Ainu custom is a great reminder that secondhand or handmade clothing is a perfectly fine choice for your baby, even if you're able to afford new items. Just keep in mind that old fabrics can carry the energies of those who once wore them, which is sometimes desirable and sometimes not. For instance, if you get a load of clothes from a thrift store and you don't know who had them before, you might want to purify and clear the clothing of any lingering energies left behind by

---

13. Anders Poulsen, *Childbirth and Tradition in Northeast Thailand: Forty Years of Development and Cultural Change* (Copenhagen: Nordic Institute of Asian Studies, 2007), 84–85.

14. Ainu Museum, "Child Rearing," in "Ainu History and Culture," www.ainu-museum .or.jp/en/study/eng11.html.

the previous owner. Just wash and dry the clothing, shake each garment vigorously, and leave the clothing out in the sun for an hour or two. On the other hand, if you happen to have an old sweater that belonged to your strong and protective grandfather, what better fabric could you find for making a little stocking cap for baby?

Hmong Soul-Calling Ceremony

Among the Hmong, an ethnic group originating in the Yangtze River basin in Southern China, an important ceremony called the *hu plig*, or soul-calling, is performed to ensure the baby's well-being. It's believed that the hu plig ceremony is necessary in order to bind the baby's spirit to his or her physical body. A name is officially conferred on the newborn baby at this time as well. The hu plig ceremony usually takes place several days after the child's birth and is often performed on the front porch or front steps of one's home. Sprigs of maple are planted in the four corners of the chosen ritual space, which are then connected with a piece of hemp twine in order to form a perimeter that will shield out evil forces. Offerings are given to the higher powers, and incantations beseeching the newborn's soul to enter the physical body are uttered by a shaman or an important family member. The name of the child is also called out at this time and may be whispered into the child's ears. Afterward, a feast is shared and everyone receives a bracelet of hemp to tie around their wrists in a symbolic act of binding the friends and family together.[15]

If this tradition inspires you, you might design your own version of a naming or soul-calling ceremony to welcome your baby. Consider inviting friends and family over for a nice meal and a celebration of your family's latest addition. You might officially announce the baby's full name at this time and invite family members to utter blessings over the baby. For the soul-calling, you might place both of your hands upon the baby's chest and, in your own words, ask the higher powers that the infant's soul take residence in the physical body, remaining strong, bright, guarded, and blessed.

15. Nicholas Tapp, "Hmong Religion," 67–68, The Chinese University of Hong Kong, https://nirc.nanzan-u.ac.jp/nfile/1512.

Brazilian Baby Booties

In Brazil, babies are given a pair of knitted booties made from red yarn. These special shoes are believed to protect the baby from evil spirits and ensure a bright future blessed with good fortune,[16] red being the color of life and energy in Brazilian culture. If you'd like to make your own lucky baby booties, choose red or another color of yarn made from natural fibers. If you're unfamiliar with knitting or crocheting, choose a simple pattern and, if possible, have an experienced crafter help you out. Before you start knitting, you might want to infuse the yarn with your well wishes and good intentions for the baby. Simply hold the yarn in your hands and think of the happiness, health, prosperity, and success you want the baby to enjoy in life. Imagine these wishes coming true, and send the good feelings in your heart out through your palms and into the yarn. If creating your own pair of baby booties seems a little ambitious, you can purchase a pre-made pair and empower them as just described; simply hold the booties in your hands as if they were the loose yarn and make your wishes.

Up Before Down for Success

One English and American folk custom is to carry a newborn baby upstairs before the baby is carried downstairs to ensure good luck.[17] This practice is believed to improve the baby's chances of achieving high status and success in life, the act seen as an effective means of symbolizing a rise in station. In the days of home births, babies were often taken up to the attic briefly. With hospitable births most common today, this tradition is heavily dependent on where in the hospital the nursery is located in relation to the labor ward, as parents typically don't have a say in such matters. You might luck out and find that your baby does indeed take the elevator up before taking the elevator down, but if not, you can still do the ceremony as soon as possible. Just think about your baby

---

16. Rebecca Gruber, "Baby Gifting Traditions from Around the World," Popsugar, July 23, 2013, www.popsugar.com/moms/Baby-Gift-Traditions-Around-World -31022688.

17. Astra Cielo, *Signs, Omens, and Superstitions* (1918; reprint, Pomeroy, WA: Health Research, 1969), 53.

growing up to be successful and respected as you carry your child in your arms up the stairs or to the top floor of a building via an elevator.

Scottish Salt Charm

In Scotland, one traditional method of conferring protection upon a newborn was to circle the infant counterclockwise with a handful of salt. This was believed to defend the baby against magickal attacks and other dangers.[18] If you'd like to do your own salt protection rite, consider performing it in an area of your home with hard floors rather than carpeting so the spilled salt will be easier to clean up. You might use sea salt, Himalayan pink salt, or ordinary table salt. Place the salt in a bowl or on a saucer. Have someone hold the baby securely in their arms. Holding the dish of salt before you, walk counterclockwise around the baby three times, sprinkling a bit of salt onto the floor as you make the circle. As you complete each rotation, proclaim that the child is protected from all dangers, shielded from all evils, and guarded from all misfortune. Sweep up the salt once the rite is complete, and dissolve this salt in a glass of warm water to neutralize any ill energies it may have absorbed. Pour the salted water down the drain.

Armenian Agra Hadig Ceremony

One Armenian ceremony called the *agra hadig* takes place when the baby gets his or her first tooth. The agra hadig is believed to help ensure the future happiness and success of the growing baby. Visitors bring gifts for the baby and share words of praise and wishes for longevity, prosperity, and joy. Special foods are served, and much singing, dancing, and merrymaking ensues. One interesting aspect of the ceremony is a custom used as a means of divining the baby's future. A selection of symbolic items is arranged in front of the baby, and the child is then carefully observed. Whichever item baby goes for first is believed to give an indication of the child's future career interests.[19] Traditionally, five

18. Rosalind Franklin, *Baby Lore: Superstitions and Old Wives Tales from the World Over Related to Pregnancy, Birth, and BabyCare* (Burgess Hill, UK: Diggory Press, 2005), 160.

19. Jim Rogan, "Armenian First Tooth," in "Local Legacies," The Library of Congress, http://lcweb2.loc.gov/diglib/legacies/loc.afc.afc-legacies.200002748.

items are used. Objects may include a book to indicate an interest in teaching, scholarship, writing, or spiritual leadership; a toy knife, stethoscope, or bandage to indicate an interest in healing and doctoring; a spoon or other cooking implement to indicate an interest in cooking; a toy hammer to represent an interest in carpentry and construction; a pair of toy scissors to reveal an interest in sewing; or some real or play money to indicate a prosperous future or a career in business, banking, or accounting.

If this tradition calls to you, you may wish to perform a similar ceremony, placing symbolic objects in front of your baby and seeing which one the child goes for first. You might include nontraditional items such as a laptop or USB drive to represent a future in technology or a CD or musical instrument to represent an interest in music. A toy airplane could represent an interest in aviation, while a pack of seeds could indicate a leaning toward gardening.

Decisions, Decisions

The moment you have a baby, you're faced with making several very important decisions, such as when exactly to cut the cord, whether to get the baby circumcised, and whether to co-sleep or let the baby "cry it out." There are also the issues of cord blood banking and what to do with the placenta.

We're not here to offer you advice on any of these decisions—believe us, you'll probably get more advice than you can stand from other people. What we want to emphasize instead is that these decisions are *your* decisions. You must do your own research and make the choices that feel best for you and your family and no one else. You can research all sides and maybe do some asking, but in the end, you need to honor your own instincts. You don't have to tell everyone about the choices you make. Many people will offer their advice on what to do and what not to do, but ultimately it is your child and your decision. Books can be contradictory, friends can be opinionated, and doctors can have biases and agendas. Investigate your options thoroughly and decide for yourself what's best. After you've gathered as much information as possible, try this simple meditation to help you get centered and in touch with your deepest feelings so you can make the very best choices:

Sit or lie down in a quiet place. Let the peace and quiet of your surroundings fill you with a sense of calm and serenity. Once you feel centered and grounded, think about the important decision you're contemplating, whatever it may be. Go into yourself and explore your feelings. What thoughts feel good and what thoughts give you an anxious feeling? Notice how the energy of your body changes as you focus on different thoughts. Once your mind has settled into a peaceful groove, think about the energies of the earth beneath you, deep underground. Envision these energies surging upward into your body. Think again of your decision. How does the earth energy seem to resonate with this choice? Does it feel in harmony with your decision, vibrating rhythmically perhaps? Or do you get a sense that something is urging you to think twice, to do a little more research possibly? Acknowledge this voice of the earth, then listen to what your heart tells you and act accordingly.

Prepare for Poo

Of course we all expect our babies to poop, but before you actually become a mother, you might not realize just how much poop you will have to deal with. On average, a newborn baby will soil ten or more diapers a day during the first month of life. That's a lot of poop, and with all that poop comes a lot of odor. There are a few things you can do to minimize the unpleasant stench of dirty diapers. For starters, whether you're using cloth diapers or disposables, shake off any solid excrement into the toilet before placing the diaper into the bin. Make sure you're using a diaper pail or garbage can with a tight-fitting lid, and line the container with a thick plastic bag. You might want to draw a pentacle on the lid of your diaper bin, using this magickal symbol to help bind in the odors and contain the stench.

All-Natural Diaper Pail Deodorizing Disks

You can further neutralize the poo and pee smells with your own all-natural diaper pail deodorizing disks. Just add twelve drops essential oil to ¾ cup water. You might use lemon, tea tree, or lavender essential oil.

Then add the water to two cups baking soda a little at a time to form a thick paste. Line a muffin tin with paper baking cups or use a silicone mold, then spoon the baking soda mixture into the cups so they are about half full. Smooth the tops and place the tin in a warm, airy place. After a day or two, the baking soda mixture will harden to form little disks that you can then pop in the bottom of the diaper pail for a boost of freshness that will last for weeks at a time. Store your diaper deodorizing disks in an airtight container away from moisture, and replace as needed.

Nursing

Whether or not to breastfeed your baby is a personal decision, and one that should be made with your lifestyle in mind. In many ways, nursing is more convenient than bottle feeding. There are no formulas to mix and no supplies to carry, and the milk is always at precisely the right temperature, right there and ready to go. At the same time, though, not every woman feels comfortable nursing in public, even discreetly. Some mothers choose to use a blend of breastfeeding and bottle feeding, while other mothers choose to stick solely with one option or the other. Not all mothers are able to breastfeed.

If you do choose to nurse, you'll need to be patient with both yourself and your baby. Nursing does not come easily for some, while it comes incredibly naturally for others. It may take a little practice before you and your baby are in sync, but if you stick with it, it will become second nature in no time. There are also lactation consultants at most hospitals, and breastfeeding classes are often offered if you feel you need some extra help and guidance. Nursing has many benefits for the baby's health, and it's good for you too. Here are some of the top reasons to consider breastfeeding:

• Nursing takes that baby weight right off you. While you shouldn't expect to become instantly thin after breastfeeding a few times, each time you nurse your baby, you're encouraging weight loss and stimulating your uterus to return to its normal pre-pregnancy size. It takes nearly a year to have a baby, and it can take just as long to regain your pre-baby figure. Nursing can significantly cut down on that time and help you get back in shape more quickly.

• Nursing lowers your risk of breast cancer. The longer you nurse, the greater the decrease in your cancer risk.

• Nursing feels amazing! It releases so many hormones and opiates in the body that you have no choice but to lie there and do nothing. You become submerged in the nursing flow, gently rocked by wave after wave of slow, gentle, really groovy feelings. Breastfeeding is designed to make the mama feel good and calm so that she will stay still and let the little one nurse until done. Nursing also provides a lot of skin-to-skin contact, which is a great way to bond with your baby. Bonding with your baby is beyond anything that can possibly be said eloquently. It just is. It is beyond. It is beauty, and grace, and nature and love and anything else loving and kind and sweet you can think of—it is.

Magickal Lactation Cookies

Your milk supply can change on a dime. If you're stressed-out, exercising too much, or wearing a bra that is too tight, your milk supply will decrease, while if you're happy, relaxed, and adequately nourished with just the right stuff, your milk supply will increase. If you're having a hard time producing milk, try getting in a little more rest and relaxation, and be sure you're eating enough healthy, nutritious food. There are three simple ingredients that, when combined, can dramatically increase your milk supply. These ingredients are raw oats, flaxseed, and brewer's yeast. Here's a handy recipe that combines these three powerhouse ingredients into one easy-to-make, magickally enchanted lactation cookie. Feel free to adapt it, but keep the proportions of those three key ingredients the same.

2 heaping tablespoons flaxseed meal

4 tablespoons water

1 cup butter or margarine, softened

¾ cup sugar

¾ cup brown sugar

2 eggs

1 teaspoon vanilla extract

2 cups flour

1 teaspoon baking soda

½ teaspoon salt

2 heaping tablespoons brewer's yeast

3 cups oats

2 cups chocolate chips (optional)

½ cup peanut butter (optional)

1 cup dried coconut flakes, raisins, or dried cranberries (optional)

Preheat oven to 375 degrees F. Mix the flaxseed meal into the water, stirring as you think of the nurturing, fertile energies of the flaxseed combining with the purifying, satiating qualities of the water. Set this mixture aside for about five minutes. Combine the butter and sugars, then slowly add in the eggs. Stir in the vanilla extract, thinking about the loving energies and magickal power of the vanilla combining with the other ingredients. Add in the flaxseed mixture once it has sat for long enough. Next, in a separate bowl, mix together the flour, baking soda, salt, and brewer's yeast until thoroughly blended. As you stir, think about the brewer's yeast causing the whole mixture to expand, just as it will cause your milk supply to increase. Mix these dry ingredients in with the wet ingredients, then stir in the oats, envisioning the strong, robust, healthful energies of the oats blending into the dough. Finally, add any additional ingredients you've opted for, such as chocolate chips, peanut butter, or raisins. As you give the mixture a final stir, visualize yourself nursing your child, imagining the milk flowing freely and plentifully from your breasts. Drop the cookies into little tablespoon-sized dollops onto a greased cookie sheet, and bake for about ten minutes. Makes several dozen, depending on the size of your cookies.[20]

---

20. Based on "Housepoet's Famous Lactation Boosting Cookies," The Breastfeeding Center, Massillon, OH, www.thebreastfeedingcenter.com/files/46628276.pdf.

More Tips for Nursing Mamas

Here are a few more quick tips to help you breastfeed successfully, conveniently, and enjoyably:

- If your nipples are sore, skip the fancy nipple creams. Simply rub them down with your own milk right after nursing. The milk will help clean any clogged ducts and is soothing to the skin.

- If it's cold at night, consider wearing a nursing shirt. You'll be able to keep your shirt on and just undo the pocket to expose your breast for nighttime feedings. If you don't want to purchase a nursing shirt, you can make your own. One of your authors here actually made a rather unattractive makeshift nursing shirt by simply taking an old thermal long john shirt and cutting out two large holes for the breasts. Ugly, yet highly effective.

- Carry a piece of malachite or pink or blue chalcedony with you. These stones are reputed to increase the milk supply and help ease any discomforts of nursing.

- Don't worry about overfeeding your baby. Your body won't produce more milk than the baby needs. You can't overfeed a breastfed baby. Your baby will want to eat when hungry, so let them.

- Put pillows on the floor. If you're breastfeeding your baby while sitting in a chair and you're feeling drowsy, place some pillows on the floor surrounding you or have your partner stay in the room with you just in case. You don't want to doze off and have baby accidentally roll right out of your arms.

- Pump now, serve later. For more flexibility and convenience, consider pumping some of your milk to store in bottles that you can use while on the go if you're going to be someplace where you don't feel comfortable nursing. Simply put the milk into sterilized, airtight containers. It will keep for to up to five days in the refrigerator and up to six hours at room temperature.

- Carry a small blanket. You never know when or where your child will want to nurse, so keep a small blanket handy so you'll have the option of privacy if you need to offer an impromptu feeding.

Colicky Babies, Oh My!

We all love our babies, but a colicky infant capable of screaming for hours on end can be challenging, most definitely. When your baby is fussy, it can be difficult to enjoy the "joys of motherhood" we hear so much about. Doctors don't agree on exactly what colic is or even if it truly exists, and effective, recognized remedies for colic are even harder to pinpoint. Colic is often used as an umbrella term to describe a baby who cries a lot for no apparent reason. There can be any number of contributing factors that lead to a fussy baby, from gas and other stomach upset to general crankiness and a need to vent frustrations. In fact, the perception of a baby as "colicky" is heavily dependent on parental attitudes. All babies cry, and what may seem like excessive crying to one parent might be considered normal crying to another.

In general, if your baby cries for more than three hours, more than three times a week, it's fair to assume that your baby cries more frequently than most other babies. There is no hard and fast rule, however. If you suspect your infant may be colicky, the best course of action is to discuss this with your doctor. Your doctor will be able to evaluate your individual situation and provide an effective strategy for meeting the needs of your family. After ruling out other possibilities such as milk protein allergies, strategies for addressing the colic may include learning a variety of techniques for soothing a fussy baby, learning coping strategies to help you deal with stress, and nurturing your ability to see through the tears to perceive your baby as positively as possible. Although colic can seem to last forever, it typically resolves on its own by the time your child is three to four months old. Knowing the end is in sight can help you to keep an optimistic, confident outlook in the meantime. You might also consider some of the following remedies.

Massage for a Happier Baby

One technique that can help relieve gas-induced colic is baby massage. When massaging your baby, use your whole flat hands. Place your hand flat on the child's belly, just below the rib cage on the left side, and move your hand in a clockwise circle. Do not go deep, but instead rub gently, moving your whole hands with love and presence in a slow and steady rhythm. Visualize a loving energy flowing out of your hands and into your baby's tiny body.

If you would like to use a massage oil, stick with ingredients that are known to be safe. Babies have very porous skin, and whatever you put on that skin has the potential to enter the bloodstream. Grapeseed oil, coconut oil, avocado oil, or olive oil are considered safe choices for external use on babies. If there is another oil you would like to use, check with your doctor first to make sure it's okay for baby. If you like, empower the oil with energies of love, comfort, and healing. Simply hold the oil in your hands and envision your baby feeling loved, happy, content, and comfortable. Send these energies into the oil to bring out its naturally occurring healing properties. Rub your baby's belly for a few minutes at a time or for however long seems comfortable for both of you.

As an alternative, try holding your baby tummy-side down across your legs. Gently sway back and forth to rock the baby. Place a hand flat on the child's back and rub gently in slow clockwise circles or rhythmic up and down movements. Pat the baby's back a few times to see if they will burp. As you do so, say, "Out, gas! Out, pain! Out, discomfort!" Many parents proclaim that a little tummy time can do wonders for a colicky baby, as this position can help relieve gas and pressure that might be causing discomfort in baby's stomach.

Another technique that might help bring baby some relief is to bend the child's knees slowly, gently, and fully into his or her chest. This little movement of rocking the knees into the chest and back out should be done very slowly (each motion is done over the course of several deep breaths). Repeat at least three to five times in a row to help calm the baby's tummy. You can also softly circle baby's knees around in each direction to help further relieve any lingering gas.

Traditional Folk Magick Remedies

You might also want to try some traditional folk magick methods of soothing colic. From stones to herbs to amulets, mothers have been warding off colic for thousands of years using time-honored magick. Just be sure to use your best judgment and put the safety of your infant first at all times; some of the older remedies are considered unsafe by today's more enlightened standards. However, it's easy to adapt a method for safety while retaining the core magick of the charm. For example, many of the older charms for colic involve administering to the infant potions containing herbs and even powdered stones. We know now what a dangerous business that can be and wouldn't dream of giving our babies any sort of home remedy like that without first getting approval from a doctor. Other charms recommend tying various stones, herbs, or amulets around your baby's neck or tummy, which is also not a good idea for obvious reasons. However, with a little common sense and creativity, we can still utilize the same herbs and stones safely and derive the same magickal benefits. Follow these simple rules for safely adapting traditional remedies:

- Never give your baby any herbs, essential oils, or powdered stones to eat or drink. Such ingredients can be toxic, so never administer any of these to baby without the express knowledge, approval, and recommendation of your doctor.
- Never tie anything around your baby's neck or other body parts. Jewelry of any type is considered unsafe for infants, as it can be a choking and strangulation hazard.
- Keep all items that could potentially present a choking hazard out of reach at all times. Do not leave anything in the crib or within reach that the baby could potentially choke on.

Utilize herbs and stones carefully. Tie the herbs or stones securely in a fabric bundle, and rub this gently across your child's skin or hold it near the body for a few moments. Put it safely out of reach once you're done. As another alternative, you might stash the bundle of herbs or stones on a high shelf or other out-of-the-way, inaccessible place in the baby's room. If there isn't a place like that in the nursery, you might keep the little bundle in your own purse or in a safe location elsewhere in your home. Just tuck a photo of your baby into the pouch along with the herbs or stones. You might also put a selection of anti-colic stones in a spray bottle filled with plain water to use as a magickal room spray to help calm baby.

Here are some modern versions of traditional colic charms to try. Just make sure to follow the previous safety guidelines.

Anise: The Pennsylvania Dutch used anise to soothe the discomfort of colic. Anise oil was mixed with mineral oil and sugar and placed on a rag for the baby to suck on. While this practice is no longer recommended, you might create an herbal charm bag featuring anise seed and place this somewhere near your baby but safely out of reach.

Amber: In the Baltic regions and in many other places throughout Europe, babies are often given amber necklaces to soothe colic and other common infant ailments. While placing jewelry on your baby is considered unsafe, you might wear an amber necklace yourself so that your infant might benefit from the proximity, or you could place some amber in your child's nursery, somewhere up high and out of reach.

Copper: In American folk magick, copper was considered the metal of choice for soothing a fussy baby. The copper was typically fashioned into a bracelet to be worn by the child, but for a safer alternative, you might place a small copper bowl or other ornament in your child's room.

Coral: The ancient Romans valued coral as a preventative for colic. Coral branches of various colors were incorporated into jewelry, highly prized for their protective and healing virtues. While you don't want your baby munching on a coral necklace, you might consider creating an anti-colic altar in your home to include a photo of your baby, some pieces of coral, and any other soothing stones, herbs, or objects that seem fitting to you. Just make sure it's all safely out of baby's reach.

Fennel: British parents often used fennel to treat their colicky babies. Fennel is traditionally brewed into a tea or syrup to be administered to the baby, which is no longer recommended. However, as a safe alternative, you could simply place a bundle of fennel somewhere out of reach but close by so that your baby can benefit from being in proximity to the plant's magickal healing energies.

Iron: In European folk magick, rings of iron were worn to soothe colic. While your infant shouldn't be trusted with a tiny ring on his or her tiny finger, you might incorporate some iron into the nursery room décor.

Jasper: The ancient Greeks used jasper amulets to help prevent colic. Upon the stone was sometimes carved an image of Hercules strangling a lion. The amulet was set in gold and worn as jewelry. Green jasper was also used. Engraved with the image of a scorpion, the green stone was set in silver and worn close to the stomach to help ease any gastrointestinal upset. While your baby shouldn't wear jewelry, you might try briefly rubbing a smooth, polished jasper stone over your baby's tummy.

Knotted String: One folk remedy for colic that flourished in the Southern United States was the knotted string. Take a string and tie seven knots in it, thinking as you do so of the infant's colic being bound up, the discomfort diminished. Traditionally the string was to be bound around the baby's abdomen, but don't do that; it's not safe. Instead, place the string up high out of reach of the baby, or carry it securely in your pocket or purse.

Take Care of Yourself

Many things will change once your baby arrives. Each baby is unique and it's impossible to anticipate the joys and challenges that your child will bring. Your baby will show you who they are over time, and through the different stages of development you will encounter various obstacles as well as wonderful moments that can't possibly be predicted.

Babies are both fascinating and time-consuming. It's easy to get so completely absorbed in your baby's sweetness and in the ongoing diaper changes, feedings, and other care duties that you forget about yourself entirely. This isn't good for you or your baby, so don't do it. Take care of yourself first so that you will be there 100 percent when your baby needs you. If you let your own energy get depleted, you'll be too exhausted to be at your best. Taking care of yourself is paramount. Here are a few simple guidelines to help keep yourself healthy and happy:

- Get plenty of rest. It's natural to need more rest than usual after having a baby, especially if you're nursing. Give yourself time to sleep and nap as much as you're able and inclined; it will help your body heal and replenish your energy.

- Continue to eat well like you did while pregnant. You know that wholesome, healthy feeling you may have felt while pregnant? A lot of that comes from pregnancy hormones, but some of it also comes from the fact that we often eat better than ever during this time of our lives. Pregnancy often prompts women to give up alcohol, tobacco, and caffeine, to cut back on sugar or cut it out entirely, and to eat a lot more fruits and vegetables and other healthy foods. Why not continue to make smart food choices for yourself now that baby is here? Don't you deserve to feel your best? While you won't need to eat as much as you did while you were pregnant, you can still make good dietary choices. Nourish yourself as much as possible by eating a sensible, healthy diet, and consider taking a multivitamin (or prenatal vitamin if you're nursing) to ensure you're getting an adequate supply of vitamins and minerals.

- Hydrate. Be sure to drink plenty of water every day. This means drinking a half ounce to an ounce of water per pound of your body weight each day. If you're nursing, you may need to drink a little more. It helps to keep a water bottle with you to sip on throughout the day.

- Wear a quartz crystal and a jade. These stones will help keep your ambition and motivation to achieve your own goals high.

- Make time for yourself. If you don't, you'll get burned out and frustrated far more easily. It's important to do something you want to do, something of your own choosing, at least once a day. This could be as simple as taking a few minutes to meditate under the tree in your backyard or taking a stroll around the block by yourself or with your dog. The main point is to get some time to yourself, even if it's only for a little bit. Let the people around you know that you need this time, and ask them for their help. If you and your baby are on your own, consider finding a trustworthy friend or neighbor who might be willing to give you a break. If you know other moms you trust, you might ask them if they would be willing to swap babysitting duties—chances are, they could use a break too. At least once a month, and more if you can manage, do something a little more extravagant, some sort of adventure just for you that takes you away for at least a good hour or two, and maybe longer. This might be a class you want to take, a concert you want to attend, a hobby you want to pursue, a talent you want to devote time to developing—anything at all of your own choosing. You might decide to use the time to go shopping, hiking, visiting with friends, or reading. Just choose something that's true to your own interests, and make it a priority to take this time for yourself regularly. Doing so will help you be a much better mom in the long run because you'll feel more refreshed, energized, whole, and fulfilled.

- Make time for magick. Keep your sense of wonder and spirituality alive by making time for magick as often as you can. Work a little kitchen magick into your cooking routine, or cast a simple charm for happiness and good luck on the necklace you're wearing. It doesn't have to take a long time to make magick a part of your daily life, and doing so will help you stay magickally empowered and spiritually in touch.

- Take time to be in nature. Try to get some fresh air every day. Put the baby in the stroller and enjoy the sights, sounds, smells, and the feel of the outdoors. Walk barefoot if you can. Gaze up at the moon and stars; notice the clouds. Doing so will help you feel more relaxed, grounded, and centered as you undergo this great transformation into motherhood.

Chapter 8

~~~~⌒ɔ·ɢ⌒~~~~

Baby Astrology

Astrology dates back to at least the third millennium BCE and is known to cultures around the world. The belief that by observing the heavens we can recognize patterns that reflect our lives here on earth is an ancient and enduring one. However, it's important to recognize that there are many different astrological systems, which are often contradictory to one another. Even if you study various systems in detail, you're getting only a glimpse of the full picture, and it may very well be a confusing one at that.

While astrology can give you hints about your child's inner nature and general disposition, it's only one way of viewing various aspects of the very complex being that is your whole child. Our personalities change and develop; our feelings and motivations fluctuate. We can no more be contained by our zodiac profile than we can be defined by words in a dictionary. There's a lot to astrology and it can definitely provide you with some valuable insights, but keep in mind that even the stars in the heavens can't possibly know it all. In this chapter, you'll get a quick overview of three different zodiac systems to gain new insights into your little baby.

Western Astrology

Based on the work of Ptolemy and having its origins in Hellenistic and Babylonian traditions, Western astrology assigns meaning to the positions of various celestial bodies at exact moments in time, such as a person's date and time of birth. In sun sign astrology, which is the system Westerners are most familiar with, only the position of the sun is considered. In this system, there are twelve signs of the zodiac, each corresponding to a month-long period of the year and associated with its own mythological figure and constellation.

Here you'll find a basic overview of the Western zodiac. Keep in mind that this information is based only on a person's sun sign. To get a fuller, more detailed picture, have your child's full natal chart done by a professional astrologer who will consider not only the date of birth but also the exact time and location of birth in making their calculations.

Elemental Correspondences

The twelve signs of the Western zodiac can be described according to elemental correspondence, with each of the four classical elements—earth, air, fire, and water—governing three of the signs. The elements are used to describe a person's general nature, or personality type. Though certainly not a hard and fast rule, signs of the same element type tend to get along well with each other, while contrasting elements (such as fire and water) may find their personality clashes challenging.

Earth (Taurus, Virgo, Capricorn): Signs ruled by the earth element are practical, loyal, steadfast, determined, responsible, and sensible. They often have a deep love of nature and they highly value realism and honesty.

Air (Gemini, Libra, Aquarius): Signs ruled by the air element are intellectual, idealistic, sociable, and unconventional. They often have an extreme fondness for adventure and are quick to make decisions and take action.

Fire (Aries, Leo, Sagittarius): Signs ruled by the fire element are passionate, energetic, impulsive, and courageous. They often crave excitement and are usually quite motivated and ambitious.

Water (Cancer, Scorpio, Pisces): Signs ruled by the water element are sensitive, emotional, dreamy, and creative. They tend to have a great love for the mystical and are often highly intuitive.

Cardinal, Fixed, or Mutable

The twelve signs of the zodiac are also grouped together into three categories called the three qualities, or modes: cardinal, fixed, and mutable. These qualities are used to describe the various motivations and general behaviors of each sign. There are four signs in each grouping.

Cardinal (Aries, Cancer, Libra, Capricorn): Cardinal signs are go-getters. They aren't afraid to try new things or be the first to do something. Always doing and striving, they're prone to overexertion and can sometimes be a little too pushy or intense.

Fixed (Taurus, Leo, Scorpio, Aquarius): Fixed signs value stability and are resistant to change. Reliable, determined, and persistent, they're willing to put forth great effort to accomplish their goals. Strong-willed and confident, they can be a bit stubborn or bossy at times.

Mutable (Gemini, Virgo, Sagittarius, Pisces): Mutable signs are flexible and adapt well to changing circumstances. Versatile, resourceful, analytical, and optimistic, they're natural problem solvers and people pleasers. They have a tendency to be easily influenced and can sometimes be very suggestible.

The Twelve Signs of the Western Zodiac

Aries (March 21–April 20): Even as tiny babies, Aries are intelligent and active, eager to meet the world and win it over with their natural charisma. Energetic, courageous, high-spirited, willful, and independent, your Aries child will love to explore and may be quite daring, so you'll have to keep an extra close eye on your little tyke. They tend to become very restless when bored, so keep them interested with a variety of stimulating sights, sounds, and experiences. Aries kids love being physically active and greatly enjoy hands-on activities and games involving lots of moving and doing. Ambitious and self-assured, they can be a little bossy at times and are easily irritated when they don't get their way. Provide them with opportunities to take responsibility and utilize their natural leadership abilities, and they will respond with enthusiasm and effort. With an innate ability to overcome even the most difficult challenges, Aries babies often grow up to be leaders, succeeding in careers as entrepreneurs, managers, overseers, and government officials, and in other positions of power.

Ruling Planet: Mars

Elemental Nature: Fire

Lucky Colors: Vibrant shades of red, yellow, and green stimulate the active Aries mind.

Lucky Numbers: 7 for Aries, 9 for Mars

Animal Totems: Ram, tiger, leopard, falcon, hawk, vulture, robin, snake, fox

Taurus (April 21–May 21): Practical yet very imaginative, Taurus children possess both the ability to dream big and the determination to realize those dreams. They love beautiful, peaceful surroundings and thrive best in harmonious, low-stress environments, so do your best to keep your home neat, calm, and aesthetically pleasing. Honest and observant, they are keen to notice even the slightest deception. Generally cheerful and mild-mannered, Taurus children attract new friends wherever they go. When their creativity is nourished, they often grow up to become accomplished artists, writers, or musicians. Dedicated and reliable, they often thrive on responsibility, so don't hesitate to give your Taurus child small chores and other duties they might enjoy. Taurus children have a strong connection with nature and will likely appreciate any chance to explore the outside world.

Ruling Planet: Venus

Elemental Nature: Earth

Lucky Colors: Subdued shades of deep blue and indigo harmonize well with the peace-loving Taurus.

Lucky Number: 6 for Taurus and Venus

Animal Totems: Bull, dove, beaver, sparrow, cow

Gemini (May 22–June 21): Gemini children are often clever, adventurous, and inventive. They thrive on the thrill of new experiences, forever questing for knowledge and adventure. Complex and dual-natured, they can appear a little moody at times, one minute happy and pleased, the next minute frustrated and irritable. Daring, intelligent, and imaginative, Gemini babies often grow up to enjoy careers in travel, communication, and the arts. They are generally very kindhearted and sensitive, affectionate, and compassionate. Geminis thrive on attention and communication, and they appreciate any chance they have to socialize or show off their many talents. Easily bored, they have a real need for novelty, so be sure to give your Gemini baby lots of opportunities to feed the senses in unexpected and exciting ways.

Ruling Planet: Mercury

Elemental Nature: Air

Lucky Colors: Pale shades of yellow, light green, silver, and white bring calm to the Gemini spirit.

Lucky Number: 5 for Mercury

Animal Totems: Dog, squirrel, deer, parrot, dolphin, seahorse

Cancer (June 22–July 22): Cancer children are very emotional, deeply loving, and acutely sensitive to any perceived injustice or show of ill will. They're careful with the feelings of others, avoiding conflict whenever possible. Though they tend to be a little on the shy and introspective side, Cancer children make excellent friends, valued for their steadfast loyalty and unwavering support of those they love. They're often very intuitive, frequently possessing strong psychic abilities. Hardworking, determined, imaginative, and extremely tenacious, Cancer children can achieve any goal they set their minds toward accomplishing, and typically grow up to attain great heights of success in their chosen career fields, often excelling in business, writing, music, and any occupation that allows them to be of service to others. They value the comforts of home and family, taking great pleasure in domestic security and family traditions. They have a deep love for nature and are especially happy around water, so be sure to provide your Cancer child with lots of opportunities to explore the great outdoors.

Ruling Planet: Moon

Elemental Nature: Water

Lucky Colors: Emerald green, white, silver

Lucky Numbers: 2 for Cancer, 7 for the Moon

Animal Totems: Crab, woodpecker, otter, seal, seagull, owl, wren

Leo (July 23–August 22): Loving, affectionate, and enthusiastic, Leo children can light up a room with their natural charm and exuberance. Proud, self-assured, and strong-willed, they love being in charge and can sometimes act a little bossy. Leos love to be in the spotlight, so be sure to give your child plenty of opportunities to show off their abilities and flaunt their talents. Generous, sympathetic, loyal, and outgoing, Leos make friends easily and are often very popular. Bold, brave, and fearless, they can be daring to a dangerous degree, so you'll need to keep an extra close eye on your young Leo. Courageous, energetic, and ambitious, Leos often achieve great success in whatever passions they choose to pursue. They often excel in careers as managers, actors, or healers and will do well in any field that allows their natural talents to flourish and shine.

Ruling Planet: Sun

Elemental Nature: Fire

Lucky Colors: Orange, yellow, gold, white

Lucky Numbers: 4 for Leo, 1 for the Sun

Animal Totems: Lion, horse, eagle, rooster, salmon, sturgeon

Virgo (August 23–September 23): Virgo babies tend to be calmer than other children of the zodiac, valuing peace and harmony above all else. They are naturally orderly and appreciate a neat, organized environment, so try your best to keep your house clean and uncluttered. They tend to have excellent powers of concentration when something interests them, and they're methodical and objective in their approach to problem solving. Flexible and accommodating, they adjust well to changes and can roll with the punches. Witty and intellectual, they often grow up to enjoy success in the literary fields, while their analytical, logical minds make them excellent scientists, detectives, and doctors as well. They can be a bit soft-spoken and introspective, so urge your Virgo child to speak up for themselves and be assertive when they have a need or an idea to express.

Ruling Planet: Mercury

Elemental Nature: Earth

Lucky Colors: Pale shades of green, blue, yellow, and gold

Lucky Numbers: 10 for Virgo, 5 for Mercury

Animal Totems: Squirrel, bear, lamb, parrot, magpie, swan

Libra (September 24–October 23): Libra babies are often easygoing and cheerful, bringing a smile to everyone around them. Optimistic, courteous, and cooperative, Libra children are easy to get along with and are able to make friends readily. They value order, harmony, and balance, so try to avoid extremes in their environments. They dislike conflict and will avoid it whenever possible, unless they determine that an injustice or unfairness has been done, in which case they will fight adamantly for what they feel is right. Imaginative, intellectual, and curious, they often grow up to enjoy an interest in science or philosophy. Fair and objective, Libras make excellent diplomats, lawyers, and judges, and they often gravitate toward careers that enable them to utilize their skills of persuasion. They love to travel and have a strong aesthetic sense, so be sure to take your Libra baby on lots of adventures to art museums, parks, and other beautiful places.

Ruling Planet: Venus

Elemental Nature: Air

Lucky Colors: Blue, purple

Lucky Numbers: 8 for Libra, 6 for Venus

Animal Totems: Hare, dove, crow, raven, owl, butterfly

Scorpio (October 24–November 22): Scorpio babies are passionate, loving, unyielding, and intense. Often attractive and filled with seemingly boundless energy, their magnetic personalities make them irresistible and highly influential. They enjoy variety and love a good mystery, and appreciate any chance to use their ingenuity and creativity. Often gifted with exceptional psychic ability and possessing a great love for the fantastic and mystical, Scorpios may gravitate toward careers in metaphysics. They also make excellent actors, as they love a bit of deception as much as they like to be the center of attention. Highly ambitious and confident, Scorpios often grow up to make their mark in the world in big, bold ways, whatever career paths they may pursue. Scorpios tend to be a bit secretive, so be sure to give your Scorpio child a reasonable amount of privacy. They have a strong need for reassurance and validation and greatly enjoy talking about themselves. Try to be a good listener and show enthusiasm for your little Scorpio's ideas and interests.

Ruling Planets: Pluto (modern), Mars (traditional)

Elemental Nature: Water

Lucky Colors: Dark red, brown

Lucky Number: 9 for Scorpio and Mars

Animal Totems: Scorpion, wolf, panther, eagle, snake

Sagittarius (November 23–December 21): Charming, caring, and fun-loving, Sagittarius babies bring lots of joy to those lucky enough to be around them. Blessed with a naturally warm and generous spirit, Sagittarius children love to share. They often have a great sense of humor and are quite sociable. They have a great love for adventure and freedom, so be sure to give your little Sagittarius plenty of opportunities for exploration and independence. Choose your battles and don't try to fence them in too tightly, as they have a natural aversion to discipline and a tremendous dislike of boundaries and restrictions. Concentration can be challenging for the Sagittarius, as they are easily distracted and often impulsive. You may have to give them extra reminders and encouragement to improve their ability to focus on a goal or task long enough to see it through to completion. Confident, optimistic, and carefree, Sagittarius children have a great zest for life and embrace everything they do with enthusiasm and energy. With their daring attitude and inventiveness, they often grow up to make successful entrepreneurs. They do well in any career involving excitement and variety, and they also flourish as educators, consultants, spokespersons, and experts of all kinds.

Ruling Planet: Jupiter

Elemental Nature: Fire

Lucky Colors: Orange, purple

Lucky Numbers: 4 for Sagittarius, 3 for Jupiter

Animal Totems: Horse, elk, falcon

Capricorn (December 22–January 20): Capricorn babies tend to be very aware and alert, yet also mellow and calm in disposition. With their patience and persistence, once they aim for a goal, they are unlikely to abandon it. Capricorn children value honesty and are unmoved by superficial flattery. Quiet and reserved, they can be a little on the timid side, so be sure to encourage your Capricorn to develop a healthy sense of self-confidence and engage in various forms of self-expression. Down-to-earth and naturally frugal, your Capricorn child will find joy in life's simpler pleasures. This sign appreciates a challenge and thrives on responsibility, so give your little Capricorn plenty of both. Industrious, hardworking, practical, and extraordinarily levelheaded, Capricorns often grow up to excel as diplomats and government officials and do well in nearly any position of management or authority.

Ruling Planet: Saturn

Elemental Nature: Earth

Lucky Colors: Gray, black, purple

Lucky Numbers: 3 for Capricorn, 8 for Saturn

Animal Totems: Goat, dog, elephant, owl, goose, deer

Aquarius (January 21–February 19): Aquarius babies are cheerful and affectionate and eager to engage with others. Acutely aware of the sights, sounds, and energies around them, they value artistic beauty and appreciate stimulating yet harmonious environments. Aquarius children are highly sensitive, so take care that you don't inadvertently hurt their feelings. They expect their emotions and thoughts to be taken seriously and can be easily offended when they feel they're being ignored or their problems are being taken too lightly. Progressive, unconventional, and often a little eccentric, Aquarius kids thrive on the opportunity to invent, create, and do things a little differently. Be sure to give them lots of opportunities to be creative both mentally and artistically, offering brain teasers, art projects, and other activities that provide plenty of space for unique expression. Intelligent, idealistic, and imaginative, they often grow up to be famed musicians, artists, and poets. They also excel as scientists, electricians, and architects.

Ruling Planets: Uranus (modern), Saturn (traditional)

Elemental Nature: Air

Lucky Colors: Vibrant shades of blue and green

Lucky Numbers: 4 for Uranus, 8 for Saturn

Animal Totems: Dog, cat, cuckoo, eagle, otter

Pisces (February 20–March 20): Pisces babies can be very psychically aware and intuitive, so don't be surprised if you and your little one seem to have a telepathic connection. Your Pisces child is likely to have an excellent imagination and may spend a lot of time daydreaming. Pisces are quick learners, having a natural knack for observing and absorbing new information. They have a tendency to be overly influenced by the opinions of others, so be sure to encourage your Pisces child to think for themselves. You may have to give your little Pisces some extra encouragement to face challenging or difficult tasks or circumstances, as they are easily discouraged. Given a comfortable, safe environment and lots of loving kindness, Pisces kids will dream big and pursue those dreams with confidence and enthusiasm. Creative, sensitive, and emotionally attuned, Pisces often grow up to be actors, artists, and musicians.

Ruling Planets: Neptune (modern), Jupiter (traditional)

Elemental Nature: Water

Lucky Colors: Lavender, purple, sea green

Lucky Numbers: 6 for Pisces, 3 for Jupiter and Neptune

Animal Totems: Cougar, sheep, ox, swan, stork, fish

Animal Zodiac

This zodiac system, based on writings by Sunbear of the Chippewa tribe and adopted and adapted by many New Age writers, reflects a combination of indigenous beliefs and modern Western astrology. It's often erroneously termed the "Native American zodiac," when in fact this particular system was not used by any indigenous tribe of the Americas. Still, modern inventions have their merits. In this system, an animal is assigned to each month-long period of the zodiac. Read on to discover more about your baby's animal sign.

Otter (January 20–February 18): Otters are eccentric, unconventional, imaginative, and intelligent. Very alert, perceptive, and intuitive, they don't miss much as they observe the world around them. Playful, dynamic, and inventive, they can be a little unpredictable at times.

Wolf (February 19–March 20): Passionate and independent, Wolves always listen to their heart and follow their dreams. Affectionate, generous, sympathetic, and loving, they make loyal companions. Sometimes they can be a little impractical and indecisive.

Falcon (March 21–April 19): Falcons are natural leaders, with an adventurous, enterprising, and persistent nature that helps them succeed in whatever they do. Open-minded and compassionate, they are very likable individuals. They can sometimes be a bit egotistical.

Beaver (April 20–May 20): Though Beavers tend to be rather inflexible and set in their ways, their strategic, methodical planning makes them one of the most efficient and effective of the animal signs. Loyal, helpful, and witty, they make reliable, trustworthy friends.

Deer (May 21–June 20): Friendly, attractive, outgoing, intelligent, clever, and blessed with a great sense of humor, Deer are a lot of fun to have near. They tend to hide their insecurities and can get restless if they feel stuck in a routine.

Woodpecker (June 21–July 21): Empathetic, caring, nurturing, and supportive, Woodpeckers are deeply emotional. Valuing safety and security, they are very protective, frugal, and resourceful. They can be rather moody at times and may have trouble letting go of anger.

Salmon (July 22–August 21): Confident, passionate, and enthusiastic, Salmon like to take a leading role in all they do. Creative, intuitive, intelligent, and generous, they tend to attract admirers wherever they go. They can sometimes be a bit conceited and arrogant.

Bear (August 22–September 21): Practical, down-to-earth, patient, and analytical, Bears are very reliable individuals who don't give up easily. Loving, generous, and modest, Bears can be a little shy, but they have a big heart underneath.

Raven (September 22–October 22): Charming, enthusiastic, and friendly, Ravens can get along well in any social situation. Patient and tolerant, they tend to be very laid-back, peace-loving, and diplomatic. Idealistic and optimistic, Ravens can be gullible at times if they don't stay on guard.

Snake (October 23–November 22): Sensitive, helpful, and perceptive, Snakes are natural healers. Imaginative and mysterious, they often develop a fondness for magick and other psychic arts. They're overly suspicious at times and tend to be rather secretive and mistrustful.

Owl (November 23–December 21): Easygoing, friendly, enthusiastic, and trustworthy, Owls have a positivity and reliability about them that makes others feel safe and happy. Daring, adventurous, and independent, they tend to feel restless rather often if not presented with enough engaging and stimulating activities.

Goose (December 22–January 19): Ambitious, determined, hardworking, and reliable, Geese never seem to rest. They tend to become workaholics or fall into obsessive behaviors if they're not careful to avoid it. Outgoing and gifted with a good sense of humor, they do know how to have fun once their goals have been achieved.

Chinese Zodiac

Each year in the Chinese zodiac system called the *Shengxiao* corresponds to a different sign exemplified by an animal. Each animal sign repeats itself once every twelve years in a continuously rotating cycle. Examining this system can help you gain new insights about your baby, yourself, and even your baby's grandparents. Take a look at the following list of animals and their corresponding personality traits.

Rat (1948, 1960, 1972, 1984, 1996, 2008, 2020, 2032): Ambitious, industrious, tenacious, shrewd, observant, clever, artistic.

Ox (1949, 1961, 1973, 1985, 1997, 2009, 2021, 2033): Loyal, reliable, determined, steadfast, hardworking, patient, honest.

Tiger (1950, 1962, 1974, 1986, 1998, 2010, 2022, 2034): Courageous, ambitious, confident, charismatic, brave, competitive, authoritative.

Rabbit (1951, 1963, 1975, 1987, 1999, 2011, 2023, 2035): Sincere, sociable, lucky, kind, cautious, skillful, peace-loving.

Dragon (1952, 1964, 1976, 1988, 2000, 2012, 2024, 2036): Lucky, eccentric, imaginative, ambitious, successful, courageous, enterprising.

Snake (1953, 1965, 1977, 1989, 2001, 2013, 2025, 2037): Intelligent, intuitive, thoughtful, flexible, wise, sympathetic, charming.

Horse (1954, 1966, 1978, 1990, 2002, 2014, 2026, 2038): Loyal, adventurous, intelligent, ambitious, witty, energetic, persuasive.

Sheep (1955, 1967, 1979, 1991, 2003, 2015, 2027, 2039): Calm, sensitive, charming, crafty, polite, imaginative, determined.

Monkey (1956, 1968, 1980, 1992, 2004, 2016, 2028, 2040): Intelligent, energetic, cheerful, confident, loyal, charismatic, inventive.

Rooster (1957, 1969, 1981, 1993, 2005, 2017, 2029, 2041): Confident, honest, energetic, kind, hardworking, organized, courageous.

Dog (1958, 1970, 1982, 1994, 2006, 2018, 2030, 2042): Loyal, courageous, intelligent, friendly, responsible, honest, kind.

Boar (1959, 1971, 1983, 1995, 2007, 2019, 2031, 2043): Determined, brave, optimistic, easygoing, honest, generous, responsible.

Chapter 9

~~~~~

Relaxation Tools for Moms

Parenthood has its perks, but let's face it: there is also a ton of stress that comes with it—especially if you let it build up. From everyday frustrations and obligations to those occasional moments of intense chaos that can make one minute seem like a million years, the pressure is bound to hit sometime or other. As a human, it's natural to experience a certain level of stress, and as a parent, it's natural to anticipate dealing with even greater stress. Not only do you have to cope with all the anxieties and challenges of your own life, but you also have to contend with the anxieties and challenges in the life of your child, this separate, precious, vulnerable person for whom you are forever responsible.

Unless you proactively unload tension before it builds up, the stress of everyday parenting can soon overwhelm you and drag you down. Suddenly, parenting situations that would otherwise be enjoyable or considered funny become episodes of panic and frustration, and before you realize what's happening, you're well on your way to losing your sense of humor as well as your mind. Don't despair! If you stay conscious of your stress level and take steps to calm yourself whenever you need to, you'll be better equipped to handle acutely stressful moments and everyday anxiety alike.

From yoga and tai chi–inspired breathing exercises, meditations, and visualizations to magickal herbs, stones, and simple rituals, you'll find in this chapter an assortment of powerful tools and effective techniques you can use to quickly calm the mind, body, and spirit. Try these techniques whenever you need to take a breather during a moment of intense stress, or utilize them every day to help maintain a relaxed and positive attitude no matter what life (or parenthood) throws your way.

Breathing Exercises for Relaxation

The breath is a wonderful indicator of your general stress level. When anxiety begins to show its ugly self, one of the first signs you'll notice is that your breathing has become short and shallow. Your shoulders begin to rise up with each breath because you feel like you can't get enough air in your lungs. You may even feel a bit lightheaded. If you notice that your breathing is becoming shallow or too rapid due to stress, take action. Being proactive about taking a moment to calm down and pause your thoughts can be a big help in keeping your breathing (and your stress level) on an even keel. Be aware of your breath, and enjoy each precious breath you take. If your breathing is too rapid, consciously focus on slowing it down. If your breathing is too shallow, consciously focus on taking deeper breaths.

There are also some really easy breathing techniques that you can do anytime, to start the day off right or to help calm you whenever you feel upset and anxious. Here are a few of the best breathing exercises to help you stay calm and centered throughout the day:

Full Yogic Breaths

Here's a breathing technique that's best utilized when you're no longer pregnant. Super easy and very soothing, full yogic breathing allows you to use 100 percent of your lung capacity. It's a perfect way to start and end your day. Lie on your back with your arms down by your sides. Keep your feet together and your legs straight. Keeping your arms straight, inhale and bring your arms up over your head until your knuckles touch the surface beneath you. Then exhale, bringing your arms straight back down to your sides. Repeat this process no less than five times, keeping your arms straight and synchronized to the speed of your breath throughout the movement.

Full yogic breaths can also be done standing straight against a wall. Stand straight with your back to a wall, your arms held straight down by your sides. Bring your heels forward an inch or so, enough to allow you to press your back firmly against the wall. Place your palms flat against the wall as well. This is the beginning position. On the inhale, bring the arms straight up overhead until the knuckles reach the wall. On the exhale, bring the arms back down to your sides. Repeat this five times.

With full yogic breathing, you are able to get the most complete breath possible without even having to think about it. Your diaphragm is responsible for 80 percent of your lung capacity. Another 10 percent comes from the chest, while the last 10 percent comes from the collarbones (clavicles.) In lifting the arms overhead, you are able to utilize all of these. When you begin to inhale with the arms by the sides, you first expand the diaphragm, then the chest, and then the clavicles. On the exhale, the opposite happens: you release from the clavicles, then from the chest, and then from the diaphragm, thus utilizing 100 percent of your lung capacity. And that's just an added bonus. When we do this exercise, we tend to focus primarily on the speed of the breath matching the speed of the arms, and this shift in attention can calm the mind in a snap.

Full Belly Breathing

If you watch a baby breathe, you will notice how high the child's belly rises with each breath. This full belly breathing is our natural rhythm, and by restoring that rhythm, even momentarily, we can reduce our stress.

Lie on your back and place one hand on your chest and the other hand over your navel. As you inhale, feel the hand on your belly rise up while the hand on your chest sits still. When we get anxious, the breath stays high in the chest. Our goal is to bring it down into the belly. Consciously breathing from the "valley" will relax your body and calm your mind. The goal is to use the diaphragm for the majority of your breathing. This means keeping the breath down low.

Fall Out Breaths

In a seated position either on the floor or in a chair, start with your arms down by your sides. When you inhale, stretch your arms out to each side and then bring them up to meet over your head. On the exhale, bring the arms back down, making an audible "ahh" sound. In using sound along with breath, you will be able to regain your sense of calm much sooner.

Yell

There is something magickal about using your voice to rid yourself of anxiety. Whether you are making a relaxing "ahh" sound or even a loud yell, there is something incredibly empowering about using your voice. When you yell, your exhale has a huge force behind it. This empties the lungs and detoxifies the body. It also releases a lot of aggression and fear. Go somewhere private where you won't be overheard, then yell, roar, or make funny sounds and see if you don't feel better afterward.

Counting Breaths

This is an easy and very helpful exercise. A lot of times when we think to breathe deeply, we think about taking a giant inhale and a little bitty exhale. Reverse that and you have a healthy, relaxing breathing pattern. Inhale for a count of four and exhale for a count of eight. In your ordinary breathing, you want the exhale to be at least equal in length to the inhale. In this exercise, it is better to make the exhale twice as long. Especially when we are feeling anxious, we do not want to think about the inhale. We want to focus on the exhale. Truly try to make the exhale long and deep. This will help your body calm itself and will take the mind out of its battle. Distraction by healthy practice is the key.

Breathe Between Your Legs

It's old-school advice that when you get nervous or feel faint, you should put your head down and breathe between your legs. The reason this idea has stood the test of time is because it has merit. When you are overwhelmed and need a little help calming down, this is a simple yet powerful trick to try. Just move your head down below your heart and breathe from this position for at least five to ten breaths. After the repetitions, wrap up the exercise by coming up slowly on an inhale, and follow up with a couple of deep, full belly breaths.

Top Ten Magickal Stones for Peace and Relaxation

Another powerful tool for relaxation comes from the earth. Stones and crystals are storehouses of natural energies, each with its own unique vibrational pattern. You can tune in to these vibrations to help settle and soothe your own internal energies whenever those stressful moments strike. Here are the top ten stones to use for staying centered, calm, and relaxed. Carry them with you throughout the day, place them around your home (out of the reach of small children, of course), or simply take a minute to hold the stone or crystal in your hand to help calm yourself whenever the need or mood strikes you.

Agate (Blue Lace, Crazy Lace, or Moss): Eases fears, relieves stress, and encourages hope and cooperation.

Amethyst: Lowers stress, restores balance, brings contentment, transforms negativity, and promotes peace.

Aquamarine: Clears the mind, calms, relaxes, eases emotional burdens, and promotes peace.

Carnelian: Clears the mind, expands perception, grounds, calms anger, and neutralizes negativity.

Howlite: Calms deep-rooted stress, balances emotions, soothes tension, and encourages relaxation.

Jet: Absorbs negativity, alleviates fear, stabilizes emotions, and brings balance.

Lepidolite: Eases the stress of transitions, alleviates stress, and promotes calm and balance.

Moonstone: Brings serenity, calms, tempers reactions, and promotes emotional healing.

Rose Quartz: Calms, soothes, restores harmony, and imparts a loving energy.

Topaz: Releases tension, relaxes, brings feelings of emotional support, and aids in resolving problems.

Using Stones for Relaxation

There are many ways to utilize the relaxing benefits of stones in your daily life. You might consider placing your magickal stones in areas of the home where stress typically occurs most often. This acts as a preventive measure to help ward off and soothe general anxiety and negativity that would otherwise build up in your living space. Be sure to keep your stones out of the reach of small children, though, as any small object presents a choking risk. You might place your relaxation stones in a potted house plant, letting a bit of the stone poke up out of the soil. Or you might arrange your stones in an attractive display in a curio cabinet, on the mantle above the fireplace, or on a high table or bookshelf. Place the stones on a rectangle of dark-colored cloth such as black velvet to help accentuate and highlight the beauty of your collection. You can even hang your stones, tying them to small lengths of cord and suspending them above windows. Just be sure the stones are securely attached so they won't fall off and become a choking hazard.

If you want to utilize the relaxing properties of stones even when you're on the go, consider wearing them on your person or carrying them with you in a pocket of your clothing or handbag. You might wear the stones in the form of jewelry, choosing a special ring or necklace pendant. You might create a special bag, placing your relaxation stones inside a small pouch or tying them up in a small square of fabric. Depending on the size of your bag, you can wear it as a necklace, or simply tuck it into your purse or pocket. By keeping your relaxation stones close to your body, you'll have access to their calming energies whenever you need them most.

Stones can be used to help you stay more relaxed and calm in general, and they can also be a powerful tool for combating anxiety in the moment. Whenever you feel you could really use a time-out, take a moment to yourself and try handling one of your relaxation stones. Place the stone on your palm and gently cup your fingers around it. Let your stress and tension pour into the stone. Envisioning the stress as a black or gray beam of light can help you to transfer your negative energies into the stone. Imagine the stress pouring out of your fingers and going into the stone. When you feel like you've emptied yourself of as much stress as possible, focus on absorbing the relaxing energies that the stone provides. Open your mind to the stone's vibrations, and allow these energies to enter into you. Concentrate on adjusting your own internal vibration to harmonize with the energetic qualities of the stone. If the stone seems to have a peaceful vibe, try to mimic that feeling. If the stone seems to have a loving energy, open your heart to receiving that love.

Using Scent to Soothe and Calm

In addition to breathing techniques and magickal stones, you can also incorporate into your relaxation arsenal the heady power of aroma. Scent is indeed magickal, able to transport our minds to other places and transform our emotions in an instant. Certain scents can help us relax, bringing a sense of peace and contentment. These scents are the stressed-out parent's best friends, able to calm, soothe, and relieve daily anxiety in a flash.

Dried herbs, fresh herbs, or concentrated preparations like essential oils are all effective mediums for making use of the magick of scent. When working with herbs or essential oils, however, it's important to be aware of potential dangers and to follow certain precautions. First off, always know exactly what you're using. This means that if you're not sure what type of herb or oil you have, or whether or not that particular herb or oil is safe to use, don't use it. Some essential oils—like pennyroyal, for instance—are downright toxic and can lead to miscarriage or other serious health complications if taken internally. Others, like cinnamon essential oil, can cause severe skin irritation in many people. Do some research to ensure that any new herb or oil you're considering is safe to use in the way you intend to use it. Also be aware that many oil preparations you'll find are actually synthetic, containing various chemical additives. Be sure to buy products labeled as pure essential oil, so you'll know exactly what's in them. Despite the necessary precautions, there are lots of ways to utilize the power of scent safely.

Here are some additional guidelines to follow to avoid any potential risks when working with herbs or essential oils:

• To err on the side of caution, never use an essential oil or other concentrated herbal preparation internally, unless specifically directed to do so by your doctor or other qualified medical practitioner.

• Avoid applying essential oils to the skin during pregnancy unless you're absolutely certain it's safe.

• If you're not currently pregnant and you want to use an essential oil on your skin, make sure the oil you choose is not a skin irritant, and always use it sparingly and in a diluted form of no more than 3 percent essential oil in a carrier oil such as jojoba or coconut.

There are many ways to incorporate the magickal power of scent into your world without having to worry about any risk of unwanted side effects and without having to do a ton of research on each specific essential oil you'd like to use. Just limit yourself to a quick sniff or two of the oil and avoid using it internally or on the skin. You might put a few drops of essential oil on a cotton ball and then place the cotton ball in a plastic bag. Whenever you're stressed, just open the bag, hold your nose about six inches above the opening, and take a whiff of the calming aroma.

You might also create a scented sachet to keep in a dresser drawer, hang in a closet, or place in your handbag or in your car's glove compartment. Just take a small square of fabric, about three inches square, and place in the center a handful of dried herbs or several cotton balls scented with essential oil. Gather up the sides of the sachet and tie up the top with a piece of yarn or ribbon to secure the bundle. Be sure to keep your magickally scented sachet out of the reach of children and pets. Whenever anxiety strikes, give the sachet a quick squeeze and enjoy the scent of relaxation. Electric diffusers are also effective, but avoid them if anyone in your household has asthma or other respiratory difficulties.

You might also choose to connect to the calming power of scent through living plants, planting a small garden of an herb or flower whose aroma you find particularly lovely.

Top Ten Magickal Scents for Relaxation

Here are the top ten scents to use for relieving stress, encouraging relaxation, and restoring calm and balance. Please note that these are intended for external use only.

Chamomile: Chamomile has a light, sweet, fruity scent. It's great for easing stress, encouraging relaxation, and promoting a sense of overall calm and balance.

Jasmine: Jasmine has a sweet, warm, floral scent. It's excellent for soothing frazzled nerves and promoting a feeling of calm and contentment. Do not use on the skin if pregnant.

Lavender: Lavender has a fresh, floral scent. It's great for calming, encouraging relaxation, purifying negative energies, restoring balance, and promoting restful sleep.

Neroli: Neroli has a sweet, floral, citrus scent. It's excellent for relieving stress, easing depression, and promoting positive feelings.

Petitgrain: Petitgrain has a light, fresh, woody, and slightly floral scent. It promotes feelings of joy, restores internal harmony, relieves tension, and eases irritability.

Rose: Rose has a very sweet, floral aroma. It's especially good for easing stress in the moment as well as soothing sadness and depression.

Sandalwood: Sandalwood has a rich, sweet, woody scent with floral undertones. Use it to ease depression, relieve anxiety, and restore a sense of grounding and stability.

Tea Tree Oil: Tea tree oil has a fresh, medicinal scent. It's excellent for relieving stress and promoting internal strength and balance.

Vanilla: Vanilla has a warm, rich, sweet scent. It's great for promoting relaxation, relieving tension, and restoring feelings of well-being.

Ylang-Ylang: Ylang-ylang has a rich, sweet, heady, floral scent. It's excellent for soothing anger, relieving stress, and easing depression.

Meditations for Relaxation

Meditation is another simple and effective technique you can use to regain your sense of calm and balance whenever anxiety strikes. By helping to manage everyday anxiety and reduce overall stress, meditation can be a great aid in maintaining a state of inner peace and contentment. You don't need prayer mats, exotic incense, or any other form of equipment to meditate, and you don't need to be a Zen master or spiritual guru in order to do it. You just need you, a quiet space, and a couple of minutes.

Meditation is whatever we make of it. It's a time when we're listening to our own greater awareness, when we take time out to simply slow down, calm down, and feel a sense of goodness and energy. Try the following meditations to get you started. Once you're comfortable with the basic process, you'll be able to formulate your own effective meditation techniques for powerful stress relief whenever you need it.

One-Minute Candle Meditation

One simple meditation to try can be performed in just a minute, so it's a great one to use whenever you need to take a quick time-out and catch your breath. To start, light a candle and sit in front of it. Focus your eyes on the flame. Allow your breathing to become slower and more relaxed. Make your breaths become rhythmic. Watch the flame as it moves, calming your body and mind as the light grows and shrinks. Enjoy a feeling of peace and calm, then extinguish the flame.

Full-Body Relaxation Meditation

Here's another meditation that will help you relax both the mind and the body. Begin by lying on your back or your side. If you like, place a pillow under your head and also under your knees. Get as comfortable as you possibly can, and do your best to minimize distractions. You may want to put on some relaxing music and light some candles.

To start the meditation, first focus your attention on your feet. Curl your toes for a moment, then relax them as completely as possible. Say to yourself, "I relax my feet... my feet are relaxing... my feet are relaxed."

Then move up to your legs, first tightening the muscles and then relaxing them. Say to yourself, "I relax my legs ... my legs are relaxing ... my legs are relaxed." Proceed in a like manner throughout your whole body, progressing from legs, to back, to stomach, to chest, to shoulders, to arms, to wrists, to hands, to neck, to head, to face, to eyes, to nose, and to lips. Next, relax your brain, lungs, and heart, envisioning a calming energy entering these areas. To finish, affirm out loud or to yourself, "I relax my entire body ... my entire body is relaxing ... my entire body is relaxed." Let your body feel heavy and limp, and allow yourself to drift off wherever your thoughts carry you. Let your mind become calm and empty. Feel your eyelids become heavy. Let your lips soften and relax. Feel how your top and bottom teeth separate slightly in your mouth and your tongue rests like a wet leaf against the roof of your mouth. If practiced at bedtime, this meditation may help you drift off to sleep.

More Quick and Easy Meditations

The following meditation techniques take only a couple of minutes at most, yet they're tremendously effective at relaxing both the mind and the body. Since these meditations are so quick, they're useful tools for helping you regain your cool and relieve stress fast in the midst of a particularly challenging moment. You might consider performing these meditations daily for general stress relief and to help maintain an overall sense of balance and relaxation:

- Sit comfortably and put on music that has a good, calm flow. Close your eyes and simply smile. See what you feel from there.
- Follow your own thoughts without judgment. Just step back and become an observer of your thoughts. Give the conscious mind a break, a mini vacation from the stress of the moment. Go beyond the mind chatter and just step away from all of your thoughts and lists you start to make in your mind of things you need to do and don't want to forget. If you need to stop and write them down, do that and then start over with this.

- Imagine yourself being bathed in a light that beams from inside you, radiating far and wide to the outside universe. Visualize this light in a color that you feel is calming or healing. White is always a beautiful, pure color, as is gold. Blue helps to calm the body and the mind. Green is for healing and so is light pink. Purples and violets are always helpful for opening the third eye and the crown of the head.

- Open your palms, allowing your hands to relax. Visualize a flow of good energy penetrating into your hands and diffusing throughout your entire body.

- Place your palms in prayer position to take yourself deeper within, or open your arms wide to receive energy and insights.

- While sitting or lying down, rub your hands from your chest all the way down your body, imagining that you are cleaning off any stress or negativity as you do so. You might also drum your hands along your body to help break up the tension.

Be willing to take a few brief moments out of each day, several times a day if you like, for a quick meditation. Parenting can be overwhelming, so allow yourself some time to step back and let go of the pressures of the outside world, if only for a short time. Meditation really is not that hard to do, and the benefits in keeping your stress level down are tremendous.

Visualizations to Calm the Mind

Visualization is another technique you can use to help reduce and manage the stress of everyday life as a parent. Visualization is the act of forming mental images or pictures, just as we do when imagining or daydreaming but with the important addition of intention and conscious focus. By visualizing what we want to occur, we activate the subconscious mind, which in turn connects to the conscious mind, directing it to act in a way that will help produce the intended result. For example, if you can visualize your daily stress as a balloon that inflates with each challenging moment and then visualize that balloon of stress bursting into oblivion or floating away high in the air above you, it can make it a lot easier to actually let go of that stress in the physical reality of everyday life. Try these simple visualization methods to help release and relieve stress in both the short and the long term.

Samskara Visualization for Undoing Negative Thought Patterns

Samskara is a Hindu word used to express the concept of "mind grooves," lasting impressions that are worn into the mind as certain thoughts, or mental tracks, are repeated. Just as a river etches its way through the landscape, so too do our thought patterns cut a path of least resistance through the physical make-up of our brains. The anxiety that comes with parenthood inevitably takes its toll and can easily become a habit if we let it, a repeating cycle as we pound into our brains the notion of how very stressed and overwhelmed we sometimes feel. This visualization will help you undo this cycle and create a new mind groove, a new samskara.

Begin by imagining your mind as a large, tangled intersection of various roads and pathways. (Readers familiar with Atlanta might picture the massive interchange known as Spaghetti Junction—a tangled mass of highways, underpasses, and overpasses, all crisscrossed and zigzagged this way and that.) Imagine now that along this confused and intertwined jumble travels a semitruck, representing your fears, your anxious thoughts, your daily stress, and the amount of negativity with which you approach your everyday challenges as a parent. Think of the deep ridges in the pathways of your mind that have resulted from this heavy truckload of stress traversing the same paths of negative thinking day after day.

Now focus your mind on a new thought, something positive and affirming, and visualize this thought as a shiny new race car. Picture that race car driving straight over any imprints, or samskaras, left on your mind by stress, and visualize new roads being formed as the old samskara is wiped away. Make sure the new thought is powerful enough to affect your mind; it must be something that elicits within you an emotional or spiritual reaction. You might try focusing on an optimistic view of the future, or create a new mind groove with a positive thought and visualization of yourself as a relaxed and calm parent, capable of anything. You can strengthen the visualization with an affirmation, perhaps stating, "I'm a relaxed, loving, and capable parent, and I'm only getting better."

Visualization for Deep, Full-Body Relaxation

For a more in-depth visualization, try this. Lie down and relax your body, beginning at your feet and working your way up to the top of your head. Once you're in a safe, peaceful space mentally, imagine that you are lying in a meadow. You are lying on your back on the greenest, softest grass. Behind your head is a giant tree, and you notice that the roots of the tree run for miles beneath the ground. This tree is majestic and the leaves are beautiful. To your side is a small stream. The water is so clean that you can see the colorful rocks and crystals lying beneath the water. The water is calm and its sounds are barely audible. As you lie there in this meadow, notice the scent of the air. With each breath you take, feel a clean, crisp, cleansing air enter your nose and fill your lungs with health and peace. With each exhale, let your body release all the stress and tension that no longer serves a healthful purpose in your body.

As you lie there in that space, notice that from the top of that tree, one leaf separates itself and begins to float aimlessly in the sky. Side to side this leaf slowly glides, making its way down to the water below. In your mind's eye, put your hand into that stream, still lying on your back. Open your palm and feel the leaf make its way into your cupped hand. Feel this leaf; pick it up and place it between both of your hands. Visualize how the leaf looks from up close and from far away. See the veins in this leaf that from far away look so simple yet are in fact so delicate and intricate. Feel the water drip between your fingers as you imagine yourself still holding the leaf in your mind's eye.

As you visualize the leaf, imagine your stress as a small speck of dirt, and place this speck on top of the leaf. Slowly place the leaf back in the water, and watch as you let it float away along with your stress. Now notice what you feel like in this exact moment. Surround yourself in a bright white light, visualizing it forming a protective bubble around you. Seal this light bubble tightly around your being so that whatever negative energies you have banished cannot return. Lie peacefully in this space for as long as you can.

When you're ready, gently begin to wiggle your fingers and toes and lift your arms over your head in a big stretch. Slowly turn onto your right side (turning that way follows the blood flow from the heart and is the softest way to get up from lying down). Stay on your right side for a moment and rest there for a few breaths. When you're ready, push yourself up into a comfortable seated position with your eyes still closed, remaining in that relaxed state.

You can end this visualization with a prayer, an affirmation, or a simple expression of thanks.

Rituals for Relaxation

Rituals are like visualizations with accompanying actions, and they can be a great tool for general stress relief. By connecting our intentional thoughts and visualizations with the power of physical action, we send a message to ourselves and to the universe at large that we are setting a new, more positive pattern. Rituals can help us externalize and release the everyday stress and woes of parenting so that the negativity doesn't build up inside and drive us to the breaking point.

Here are some simple rituals to try to help you let go of stress and embrace a more positive attitude whenever you're feeling especially grumpy or frustrated.

Banish the Bad and Grow the Good Ritual

Here's a simple ritual you can use to help you embrace the positives of parenthood and release any negative thought patterns that hinder your ability to maintain a feeling of calm and contentment. Take out two pieces of paper. On one piece write the word "Embrace," and on the other write the word "Release." On the Embrace page, write down all the affirmations you can think of that express your greatest joys of being a parent. These might be statements like "It makes me happy to see my child play and grow" or "I take good care of my children and myself." On the Release page, write down all of the negative feelings that you are willing to release or that you desire to release. Be brutally honest with yourself. Your Release page might include statements like "I fear I'm no good at parenting" or "I feel like I sometimes get overly stressed about relatively petty frustrations." Mother guilt can be a serious source of stress, and it's important to address it so you can get past it. As parents, we're bound to make some mistakes, and the only thing that can be done about those mistakes is to make it right and move forward. Whatever you want less of in your life, note it on the Release page, and whatever you want more of, place on the Embrace page. When you're finished, take the Embrace page and bury it somewhere in the earth, visualizing the positive energies represented on the page as seeds that will grow and flourish. Take the Release page and shred it or burn it. As you do so, visualize the negativity and stress represented therein disintegrating along with the paper.

Bubble Ritual for Relaxation

Here's an easy and fun ritual that will help you release stress while nurturing your own inner child. You can even share this ritual with your kiddos, if you like. All you need is a bottle of bubbles. Go to a pretty place outdoors, take a few deep breaths, and start blowing bubbles. As you blow each bubble, let go of any stressful, fearful, critical, negative, or cynical thoughts. Let each bubble surround and trap those negative energies, and feel your heart grow lighter as you watch those bubbles drift up and away. If you like, you can strengthen this ritual with a simple affirmation: "I am free to let go of stress. I am free to be joyful and lighthearted. I am free to shine like a child."

Relaxing Bath Ritual

For this simple yet highly relaxing ritual, all you'll need to do is take a bath. Place ¼ cup sea salt in the water as the tub fills. While you bathe, imagine that all your stress, worry, and irritability is flowing out of your body and into the water. It may help to visualize this negative energy, seeing it in your mind's eye as a tinted light radiating from your skin. Get out as much stress and anxiety as you can, letting it flow out freely until you have a sort of "empty" feeling.

Now take a few moments to just sit in the tub and relax. Breathe slowly and deeply, letting your mind drift. When you're finished and it's time to drain the bathwater, envision all the stress and negativity you released flowing down the drain and out of your life along with the dirty water. Rinse the tub and dry yourself thoroughly.

You've Got This

Although there's no one-stop, all-powerful solution to stress management, by applying the tools and techniques in this chapter, you'll be much better equipped to handle the everyday challenges and anxieties of parenting. Relaxation is elusive for the average parent, but if you make a point of it, it's entirely possible to achieve it. The next time stress strikes, remember that you're now armed with many magickal tools and practical techniques for relieving anxiety and restoring a sense of calm both in the moment and in the long term. Without a doubt, parenting is often stressful, but as long as you don't let that stress get the better of you, the joys of taking care of a child far outweigh the challenges.

Chapter 10

~~~ 🙠 ~~~

Energizing Techniques for Moms

With constant diaper duties, baby-soothing duties, homework-helping duties, cooking chores, cleaning tasks, and everyday work to deal with, it's no wonder many mothers struggle to keep their energy levels up throughout the day. Motherhood can be absolutely exhausting, no matter how good at it you are. In this chapter, you'll learn some simple exercises and discover stones, scents, colors, and charms to help you recharge your batteries whenever you're slumping.

Energizing Rituals and Visualizations

We mothers know that just because we need a break doesn't mean we can always take one. Sometimes there are pressing demands that require our effort and attention, regardless of whether we have the energy to do a proper job of it. Whenever you find yourself struggling to ward off exhaustion or apathy and conjure up some motivation, try any of these fast and easy rituals or visualizations to increase your energy. Each can be completed in less than five minutes, and you'll be able to return to your day with a renewed sense of power and purpose.

Smiling Visualization for Energy

This visualization is super quick and easy and can be performed almost anywhere. Sit or stand comfortably, close your eyes, and simply smile. Let your feelings carry you, and allow images to form naturally in your mind. Do not stop smiling. This is the key to tapping into the energy reserves inside you. Smiling triggers a sense of gratitude and fills your mind with images of people and things you love, which in turn helps you feel genuinely happy and energized. Let these images of the people and things you love develop as fully and clearly as possible in your mind and heart, and allow those loving feelings to expand throughout your body. Grin even bigger for a moment as these feelings and images flow through you. Open your eyes and let the warmth in your soul carry you throughout the rest of the day.

Animal Power Energizing Visualization

Think of an animal you admire, something fast, fierce, strong, or courageous. You might imagine a lion, an eagle, or any other animal you feel drawn to at the moment. Visualize yourself transforming into this animal. Imagine your body changing, your mind becoming primal and animalistic. See yourself traveling easily through the wilderness, racing along the forest floor, or soaring high above in the sky. Imagine that you're looking through the animal's eyes. What does the world look like from this new perspective? If the animal you have chosen makes sound, make this sound now—roar, bark, hoot, whatever it is. If your animal is silent, take a moment to move your body like that animal. You might imagine that you are extending sharp claws, that you are spreading wide wings, that your limbs are strong and supple. Come out of your animal visualization gently. Envision yourself slowly changing back into human form. Look at the ground at your feet and see a small stone statue of the animal whose form you just took. Pick up this statue, place it in your pocket, and return to reality. By stirring up your animal instincts, this ritual will have you feeling powerful and energetic in no time.

Tree Dance Energizing Ritual

Go outside and place your hands around the trunk of a tree. Try to clear your mind and focus on feeling the energies pulsating within the tree. Get in tune with this power; feel it, listen to it, mimic its vibration with your own energy that flows from your hands. Envision a circuit of power, your energy flowing into the tree and the tree's energies flowing back into you. Absorb this energy through your hands and feel it travel up your arms and spread throughout your body, bringing a feeling of warmth, strength, renewal, and power. When you feel like your energy levels have been restored, release your grip and dance around the tree for a moment. Clap your hands together a few times while feeling the energy within you rise even further. When you feel your whole body pulsating with energy, envision your goals for the rest of the day being met with ease. Raise your arms up to the sky and wiggle your fingertips to release your wishes into the universe. Take a moment to appreciate the tree as well as the surrounding environment and express your gratitude, then return to your day with renewed power.

Energizing Water Ritual

Pour a glass of fresh, cool water. Use a clear or blue glass if possible so it's more in tune with the water element, or choose an orange or a red cup to symbolize energy. Hold the glass in your hands and envision a raging river, a rushing waterfall, or crashing waves. Call into the glass the energies of this raging water. Think of the strength and power of water, how it can cut a path through solid rock or erode away a mountainside. Imagine the water in your glass sharing this same strength and power; visualize it pulsating with a bright, clear, purifying energy. Drink the water and let this new energy flow through your body to revitalize and refresh you.

Energizing Ritual Bath

When you have a little more time to spend, try this energizing ritual bath. Cut a small circle of lace or other gauzy fabric, about three inches in diameter. If you don't have such a fabric, you can snip off the toe from a pair of old pantyhose and use that. Place on the fabric one piece of citrine, one clear quartz crystal, and a few pieces of orange peel. Gather up the sides of the fabric and tie it securely at the top to make a little bundle that will keep the stones and the orange from slipping out into the bathtub. Fill the tub and place the fabric bundle in the warm water. As you begin your bath, think of the energies of the stones and the orange blending with the energies of the bathwater. Visualize the water glowing with a bright, hot light. Think about the energy in the water and imagine this energy flowing into your body, absorbed through your skin. Trust in your abilities and pull this energy into your core. Finish your bath with a quick rinse in cool water.

Top Ten Stones for Energy

These stones can be utilized to gain a quick burst of energy when you need it most or to keep your power levels up consistently throughout the day.

Amesite: This stone increases physical energy while infusing the mind and spirit with a blast of optimism and positive power.

Aragonite: This stone increases mental confidence, replenishes physical energy, and empowers the spirit to take effective action.

Azurite: This stone is useful in bringing strength, increasing tenacity, and activating the unused power of your mind, body, and spirit.

Citrine: This stone has a strong, vibrant energy associated with the sun. Use it to lift your spirits and energize your body and mind.

Clear Quartz: A natural amplifier and storehouse of energy, clear quartz can be used to activate your hidden energy reserves and give you a boost of power when you're feeling worn out.

Kyanite: This stone activates your body's energy centers and improves the flow of energy throughout the body.

Red Jasper: This stone will help fortify and strengthen your tenacity while replenishing your energy reserves.

Tiger's Eye: This stone increases physical energy while bolstering courage and boosting confidence.

Tourmaline: This stone increases physical energy and boosts mental alertness.

Zincite: This stone activates the chakras and restores your body's natural energy.

Using Stones for Energy

There are many ways to utilize stones to help increase and maintain your energy. Try placing your energizing stones in areas of the home where you find yourself feeling the most worn out. You might place them near the washer and dryer or other chore areas, or place them near your favorite resting spot—perhaps near that big, squishy chair you tend to collapse in whenever exhaustion gets the better of you. You might also carry some energizing stones in your pockets or purse or incorporate them into jewelry so they'll be near your body at all times. You might decide to keep your energizing stones in a special box and just take them out when you need them. For most of us, our energy levels tend to fluctuate throughout the day, and there are certain times when we're nearly always tired. This might be early morning for some people, evening for others, late night after the children finally fall asleep, or any time in between. You might try pulling out your energizing stones during these down times to give yourself a boost of power.

To activate your energizing stones, simply hold the stone in your hand and close your fingers around it. You might even lie down for a moment and place the energizing stones on your chest, right on top of your solar plexus, or breastbone. Feel the way the stone pulsates with energy, and envision this power being drawn into your body, filling your being with invigorating vibrations. Once you've absorbed all the energy you can from the stone, seal the deal with a positive affirmation: "I am energized, alive, awake, and great!"

Top Ten Scents for Energy

The magick of scent can help increase your energy and restore your vigor whenever exhaustion strikes. You can use scents in the form of essential oils, fresh or dried herbs, potpourri, or scented products like lotions or soaps. Remember to use essential oils sparingly and never take them internally while pregnant (and even if you're not pregnant, you must still exercise great caution to make sure what you're taking is safe). If you're using essential oil on the skin, make sure it's an oil that's safe to use that way, and be sure to dilute it first in a carrier such as jojoba or coconut oil using a proportion of no more than 1 to 3 percent essential oil. For safest use, combine a few drops of essential oil with about two ounces of water, and use it as a room spray to add a light fragrance, or simply place a drop of the oil onto a cotton ball and take a quick whiff.

The following scents can be used to provide a burst of energy whenever you need it.

Basil: Fresh and earthy, basil improves the mood and increases stamina. Attuned with the planet Mars, it works well for bolstering willpower and encouraging optimism whenever your energy level or general outlook hits a downward slump.

Bergamot: This sweet citrus scent associated with the planet Mercury and the air element has floral notes to help elevate your spirit and invigorate and recharge your mind. Do not apply directly to the skin, as it can cause photosensitivity.

Cinnamon: Rich, earthy, and spicy, the scent of cinnamon boosts energy and magnifies passion. Attuned with the fiery sun, it's a good scent to use to help you meet the day with enthusiasm and courage. Do not apply directly on the skin, as it can cause irritation.

Frankincense: This exotic, heady scent will leave you feeling strong, fortified, and spiritually attuned. Corresponding to the sun and the fire element, it's filled with powerful energies that pack a punch.

Grapefruit: The light citrus scent of grapefruit increases optimism and uplifts the spirit. Attuned with the sun, it can be used to restore good feelings and high energy when you're feeling low on power. Do not apply directly to the skin, as it can cause photosensitivity.

Lemon: Light and fresh, this scent invigorates and purifies the aura. It's attuned with both the sun and the moon and can be used to increase your energy and refresh your spirit night or day. Do not apply directly to the skin, as it can cause photosensitivity.

Marigold: This distinctive floral scent has an intensity that amplifies magickal power and replenishes an exhausted psyche. Attuned with solar energies, marigold can be used to promote happiness and recharge your inner charisma whenever you're feeling mentally drained.

Orange: Powerful and refreshing, this scent increases energy and awakens inner strength and confidence. It's attuned with the sun and is beneficial for improving stamina and encouraging cheerfulness. Do not apply directly to the skin, as it can cause photosensitivity.

Patchouli: Rich and heady, this scent magnifies passion and fortifies the spirit. Attuned with the earth element and the planet Saturn, it's a good scent to choose for grounding and centering your energies when you feel weary or scattered.

Tangerine: This rich citrus scent enlivens and cheers. Attuned with solar energies, it's a good scent to use to bring energy and improve your mood. Do not apply directly to the skin, as it can cause photosensitivity.

Colors for Energy

Incorporate these colors into clothing, jewelry, décor, and magickal charms to increase your energy throughout the day. You might try a simple color meditation, focusing on any one of the colors listed here. You can gaze at a small square of paper in the chosen color or simply close your eyes and imagine the color. Let the color flood your mind, and allow your feelings to flow naturally. How does this color make you feel? What thoughts and emotions does it inspire? Try a few different colors to find your best energizing shades. Once you have your best match, it's easy to conjure up this color in your mind whenever your energy levels could use a boost.

Gold: Spiritual strength, faith, enthusiasm, and the power of the stars.

Orange: Willpower, desire, energy, and the powers of the fire element and the sun.

Red: Passion, power, strength, and the power of the fire element.

White: Purity, energy, power, and the renewing force of nature.

Yellow: Action, swiftness, mental alertness, and the powers of the air element and the sun.

Energizing Exercises

Getting the body moving is one of the best ways to stimulate blood flow and increase your energy. Try these quick and easy exercises anytime you need to wake up a bit. These exercises are good throughout pregnancy and beyond. You might want to try doing all of these first thing in the morning to help you start the day alert and ready to go. Throughout all these exercises, keep your knees soft and keep your breath deep, full, and even.

Hip Energizer

Wake up the hips. Stand with your feet shoulder width apart and place your hands on your hips. Move your hips around in a wide, full circle, ten times in one direction and then ten times in the other direction.

Knee Energizer

Place your hands above your knees, with legs bent. Keeping your feet stationary and your legs bent throughout the exercise, move your knees around in a full circle. Go ten times in one direction and then ten times in the other direction.

Ankle Energizer

Hold on to the back of a chair or another sturdy object to help you keep your balance. Lift one foot off the ground and move your ankle around in a complete circle. Do this for ten rotations, then switch feet and do ten more circles with the other ankle.

Shoulder and Chest Energizer

Start by reaching out in front of you, holding your arms straight and spreading your fingers wide (figure 16a). Keep your knees soft; don't lock them. Pull back as if you're trying to touch your shoulder blades together, bending your elbows as far back as they will go (figure 16b). Next, swing the arms back up in front, and this time, cross one arm over the other (figure 16c). From there, swing the arms straight back (figure 16d). Now repeat, but when you cross the arms, change which arm is on top. This is all done with a smooth, swinging motion. Do this at least ten times to open up the chest, lungs, and upper back.

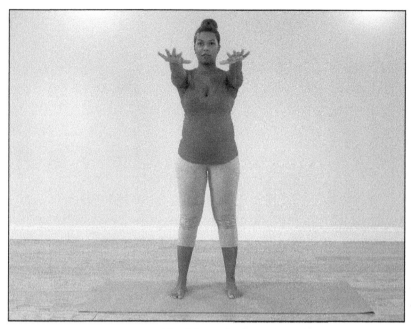

Figure 16a: Shoulder and Chest Energizer

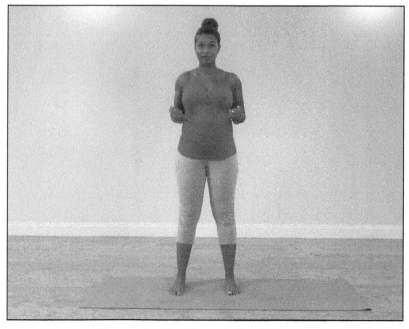

Figure 16b: Shoulder and Chest Energizer

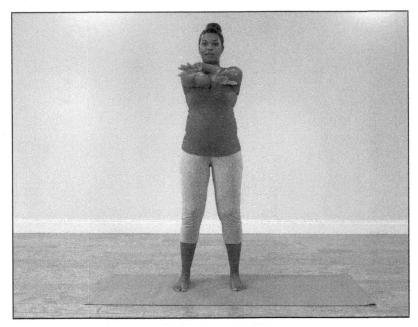

Figure 16c: Shoulder and Chest Energizer

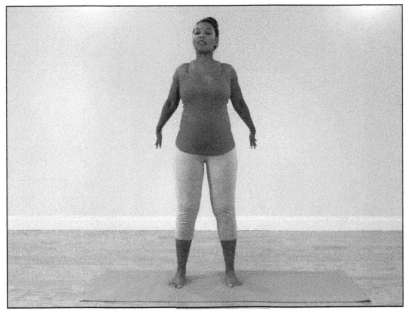

Figure 16d: Shoulder and Chest Energizer

Stimulating the Chi

This exercise stimulates the *chi*, or energy, of the entire body. Chi is our vital life force. Doing this exercise is highly effective for stimulating the chi and activating the entire energy of the body. Begin with your knees soft and your arms held loosely by your sides. After that, it's all swinging motions. To begin, swing both arms to the left side and look over the left shoulder. Next, swing your arms around to the right side, and turn your torso so that you're now looking over your right shoulder. Each time you repeat this, swing the arms a little bit higher, first level with the waist, then the ribs, then the chest, and then the shoulders (figure 17a), then returning back to the waist in descending order (figure 17b). Repeat this pattern until you achieve a steady flow of energy as you swing the arms from side to side. Keep your arms heavy and swing them like you would swing the arms of a rag doll.

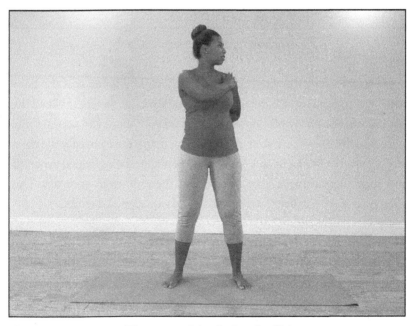

Figure 17a: Stimulating the Chi

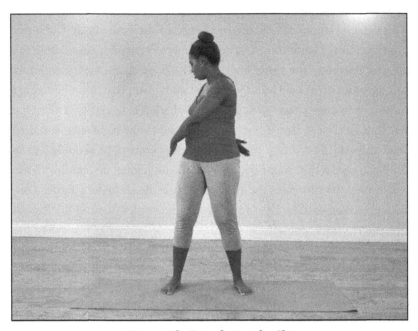

Figure 17b: Stimulating the Chi

If you're doing this exercise while pregnant, you'll find that the baby loves this movement. Be soft with your body and let the energy lead the way. Finish this off by placing your hands on your chest and taking some deep breaths. As you exhale, rub your hands down the front of your chest and stomach, visualizing any tired, weary energies being wiped away off the body. Repeat this at least three times, then return to your day. This exercise is sure to deliver anytime you need a quick pick-me-up.

Energy Every Day

You've explored many techniques throughout this chapter for increasing your energy, from simple physical exercises to stimulating scents, colors, stones, and visualizations. The only keys you need to activate these tools are sleep and adequate nutrition. If you're not sleeping well or eating right, your body has no chance of being at its best. Give yourself the rest you need and choose wisely what you eat. Combined with the tips in this chapter, you'll have a winning system to help you meet each day head-on and full of energy.

Chapter 11

~ ᧬ ~

Bathtime Magick

Bath time provides a fun and enjoyable opportunity for your baby to explore the water. While some babies take to the water immediately, others may be wary at first but will grow accustomed to the bath through regular experience. In this chapter, you'll learn some ways to incorporate a little magick into the bath routine to help your wee one get the most out of their time in the water.

Crystal Baths for Babies

There are lots of ways to bring a little magick into baby's bath. While using essential oils or heavily scented soaps and shampoos in baby's bath can be risky, increasing the chances for a urinary tract infection, rock crystals can be used to enchant a tub full of water in seconds without any potentially harmful effects. Simply choose a crystal whose magickal properties you would like to impart to the bathwater. Pick one that is medium-sized and easy to hold on to. Fill the tub, keeping the water level low and the temperature safe, and waft the crystal through the water. As you do so, envision the water harmonizing to the vibrations of the stone. Take the crystal out of the water and stow it away safely out of reach. Your baby's bathwater is now imbued with the crystal's magickal properties. Try the crystals described here, or choose your own to create unique energetic effects.

Amethyst: Healing, calming, wisdom, spirituality, and dreams.

Citrine: Happiness, purity, renewal, warmth, and energy.

Clear Quartz: Clarity, spirituality, power, insight, and balance.

Rose Quartz: Love, joy, peace, contentment, and healing.

Smoky Quartz: Strength, protection, and absorbing and neutralizing negativity.

"Drawing" a Bath

Another technique you can use to make bath time magickal is to charm the water by drawing symbols in it. Choose a symbol that corresponds to the magickal property or effect you're going for. Keep this meaning clearly in mind as you use your index finger to trace the symbol in the bathwater. Imagine the water in the tub vibrating with the magickal energy carried within the symbol until all the water seems to resonate with the properties desired.

Try the following symbols, or create your own designs to represent your loving wishes for your little one.

Flower: Happiness, beauty, playfulness, growth, abundance, discovery.

Heart: Love, comfort, peace, contentment, calming, healing.

Leaf: Nature, vitality, strength, nurturing, balance, unity.

Moon: Dreams, solace, wisdom, introspection, soothing, psychic connection.

Pentacle: Abundance, health, hardiness, luck, protection, grounding.

Sun: Joy, warmth, energy, enthusiasm, vitality, growth.

Soothing Sounds for Baby's Bath

Adding music or other sounds to your baby's bath time can make the experience more interesting, more emotionally soothing, and more mentally stimulating, and can also help establish a bathing routine that baby will come to expect and enjoy. If you don't have a waterproof music player, play the music from an adjacent room or use a non-electronic music maker. Consider the following sounds to soothe and enchant your baby during bath time.

Classical Music: Try classical composers like Mozart or Vivaldi to help calm your baby in the water and stimulate your child's mental faculties.

Music Box: An old-fashioned wind-up music box is perfect for a bath, since it's not electronic and won't be a danger if it gets wet. Music boxes generally play very soothing and uplifting melodies that will help make bath time more enjoyable for you and baby.

Ocean Sounds: Consider a CD of ocean sounds to bring a touch of nature to the bath. The sound of rolling waves and seagulls will help soothe your baby and make the bath seem like an outdoor adventure.

Wind Chimes: Hang a set of wind chimes from the bathroom ceiling. Before you put your child in the bath, hold your baby close and invite them to make the wind chimes jingle. Do the same when you take your baby out of the bath. The merry tinkling sound will help baby associate happy feelings with bath time.

Bathtime Color Magick for Babies

Color magick is another way you can make baby's bath time more special. Try choosing the towel or washcloth based on color. Just select a color that has the magickal attributes you're going for. To get the towel or washcloth ready for use, hold it in your hands and think about its color. Think about the magickal properties of that color. What energy do you want to bring to the surface? What effect are you going for? Set your intention and send those wishes into the towel or washcloth. The magickal energies will be transferred to your sweet little babe whenever the washcloth or towel touches the child's skin. Try the following color choices, or experiment with different shades.

Black: Protection, strength, solace, and banishing stress or other unwanted energies.

Blue: Wisdom, happiness, comfort, peace, and love.

Brown: Stability, balance, strength, security, and coziness.

Gray: Neutralizing negative energies, balancing chaos, and tempering intense emotions.

Green: Vitality, nurturing, soothing, healing, and luck.

Maroon: Strength, energy, love, and health.

Pink: Love, joy, calm, friendship, and kindness.

Purple: Spirituality, psychic connection, dreaming, and lunar energies.

Turquoise: Playfulness, cheerfulness, optimism, hope, and cooperation.

White: Purity, innocence, peace, and protection.

Yellow: Happiness, energy, warmth, intelligence, and communication.

Bathtime Color Magick for Older Kids

To make bath time more magickal for older children, try tinting the water with nontoxic, non-staining color tablets. Think of the color's magickal attributes spreading throughout the water as you fill the tub. Your child might also enjoy colorful crayons made especially for the bath; just ask any retailer that sells bath products. Try the following colors, or mix to create your own unique shades.

Blue: The color of the sky and the oceans, blue is a calming, expansive color that helps children let go of stress.

Green: Reminiscent of the grass and the trees, green helps children feel relaxed and nurtured in the bath.

Orange: Intense and energetic, orange helps invigorate, motivate, and excite children when they're feeling bored or lethargic.

Pink: Soft and pretty, the color pink makes for a soothing, healing bath that helps improve the mood and encourage peace after a frustrating day.

Yellow: Warm like sunshine, yellow lifts the spirit and encourages happiness as your child bathes.

Top Seven Magickal Scents for the Bath

Aromatherapy can do wonders to lift the spirit and soothe the soul, and bath time offers an excellent opportunity to discover what the power of scent can do for your child. From calming to cheering, there is truly a scent for every occasion. Simply experiment with different scents and notice which fragrances your child seems to respond to the best.

The age of your child will determine the methods you might use to incorporate the power of scent into the bathtime routine. For older children, you can use scented bath products or simply add two to three drops of diluted essential oil to the water, given your child doesn't have sensitive skin and isn't prone to urinary tract infections. As an alternative, you can cut off the toe end of a pair of pantyhose, fill it with dried herbs, tie it securely, and place it in the water to add fragrance to the warm bath. For younger children and babies, you can place a sachet of dried herbs in the bathroom (but not in the bath itself), or put a drop or two of diluted essential oil on a cotton ball and stash it out of reach on the bathroom counter during bath time. Try utilizing the following scents for a little bathtime magick.

Apple Blossom: Relaxation, contentment, happiness, love, friendship.

Coconut: Dreams, relaxation, psychic connection, love.

Lavender: Peace, healing, relaxation, comfort.

Orange: Happiness, energy, enthusiasm, courage, success.

Rose: Beauty, love, healing, calming.

Vanilla: Solace, love, psychic connection, luck.

Watermelon: Lightheartedness, contentment, kindness, friendship, play.

Taking the Chaos out of Bath Time

The main key to avoiding bathtime chaos is preparation. Have all your supplies ready, have a towel at hand, and get the tub completely ready before you bring in your little one. Make things easy on yourself by slipping on a bathrobe over your clothes, which are bound to get wet. Bath time can be filled with intrigue, magick, and fun. Try out the ideas in this chapter, or come up with your own unique ways to make your child's bath a splashing success.

Chapter 12

~~ ୨·ୢ ~~

Bedtime Magick

What mother hasn't wished for a little bit of magick when coaxing her young ones to drift off to slumberland? Even the tiniest tykes can be incredibly strong-willed when it comes to their sleeping habits and preferences. You'll have to retain a level of patience and flexibility if you want to keep your sanity. Nighttime can be scary for little ones, so be prepared to rock, cuddle, hold, or whatever it takes, whatever the hour. Face the fact that you will lose a lot of sleep with a new baby in the house, and realize also that the battle will merely change forms as your baby grows into a child. That said, there are indeed certain tricks you can use and charms you can employ to greatly increase the chances of your kiddo getting a restful night's sleep filled with happy, pleasant dreams. In this chapter, you'll learn some ways to banish bad dreams, encourage sleepiness, give a relaxing massage, and more.

Sleepy Scent Magick

Scent is a powerful tool for inducing relaxation and encouraging sleepiness. Try blending eight drops of essential oil with one cup of water to create a room spray. Spritz it a few times toward the center of the room, and add a quick spritz to the pillow or bedsheets if you like. Just be sparing in your use of essential oils around children and even more sparing around babies, and avoid it altogether if your kid has allergies, skin sensitivities, or breathing difficulties. For a lighter scent, try placing a few drops of essential oil onto several cotton balls, then place the cotton balls in your vacuum's canister so that when you vacuum the room, a faint trace of the scent will be left behind. For younger children and babies, you might consider anointing your shoulders or neck with a drop or two of diluted essential oil so your child will pick up the sleepy scent when you get close for a bedtime hug or cuddle. Try the following scents to help your kids feel drowsy and at ease when it's time for bed.

Chamomile: This herbaceous, slightly floral scent reduces agitation and relaxes the senses.

Geranium: This fresh, sweet, floral scent promotes harmony, peace, and tranquility.

Lavender: This light, airy scent encourages happiness, soothes the nerves, and promotes sleepiness.

Rose: This sweet and heady floral scent encourages feelings of love, serenity, and contentment.

Vanilla: This rich, warm scent soothes and relaxes to promote deep, peaceful sleep.

Circle of Sleepiness Charm

Cast this charm to fill your child's room with an aura of sleepiness that will help make your tot feel drowsy. Stand in the center of the room with your dominant arm extended in front of you, palm facing the wall and fingers extended. Take a few deep breaths to get yourself feeling calm and centered. Feel your inner strength and personal power welling up inside you, and imagine that you are projecting this energy through your extended arm and out through your palm into the room surrounding you. It might help to visualize this energy as a shining golden or white light. As you project the energy out through your palm, slowly rotate your body in a clockwise circle. Imagine that the energy you are projecting is pushing any stale, negative, anxious, agitated, or otherwise undesirable energies out of the space as you turn. When you get back to your starting point, close your eyes and imagine the most comfortable bed your mind can conjure. See yourself resting in this bed. Take long, slow breaths; breathe as if you were sleeping deeply. Let that drowsiness wash over you.

Spread both of your arms out wide in front of you and imagine the sleepiness you feel flowing out of your body and seeping into the surrounding room. Think of teddy bears, soft pillows, warm blankets, and a mother's hug, and let those sleepy thoughts pour out of you. Visualize the room being completely engulfed in a giant orb of sleepy, drowsy energy. It may help to picture this orb as a fuzzy pink light.

Finally, let out a big yawn, making it sound as real as possible. Get your child in the room as soon as possible after casting the charm, or put your child in the room first and let them watch you do it. Be aware that this charm can be a little too effective sometimes and you might end up making yourself sleepy in the process. To perk yourself up after the charm is cast and the kiddos are slumbering, blink your eyes quickly, shake your arms and hands vigorously, move your body around, and drink a glass of water.

Best Colors for Sleep and Relaxation

Consider these colors for room décor, walls, furniture, bedding, or sleepwear to help your child rest easier.

Green: Nature, earth, vitality, and growth. From pale sea green to vibrant shades of forest green and emerald, green is comforting and nurturing, making for a good night's rest.

Pale Blue: Water, sky, boundlessness, clarity, and purity. Like a clear river reflecting the sky on a warm summer day, pale blue is a relaxing, happy color to help put your child at ease.

Pale Yellow: Sunshine, light, intelligence, and cheerfulness. While bright yellow can be overly stimulating, shades of very pale yellow can provide just the right amount of sunny warmth to help your child feel calm and content as they drift off to dreamland.

Silver: Moonlight, spirit, mist, and dreams. Like the silvery moon, this color enchants and soothes to help entice your tot into a peaceful slumber.

Sleepytime Massage

Massaging your little one will help them relax and fall asleep sooner. Unlike adults, babies need a minimal amount of time to feel great results from massage. Try these soothing moves and your baby will be snoozing before you know it. Remember to use your whole, flat hands when massaging baby, and don't press too hard or too deep. Be gentle with your caresses. Babies seldom stay still for more than a few minutes, so the movements should be long and repeated only a few times.

As you massage your baby, visualize a comforting, loving energy flowing from your hands and into the child. If you choose to use a baby-safe lotion or oil, this is an ideal time to apply it. Hold your baby's foot in one hand, and with your other hand, rub up the leg and circle back down. Do the same with the arms, holding baby's hand in one of your hands and rubbing up to the shoulder, then coming around the shoulder and back down to the wrist. Do not put lotion or oil on your baby's hands because they will immediately rub their eyes with it.

Next, give your baby a brief belly rub. Moving your flat hand in widening clockwise circles, start small around the navel and widen the circle until you reach the ribs. Be gentle; do not press deeply at all. Next, rub up the chest and out to each shoulder. You might even stroke baby's face a little, tracing the eyebrows, nose, and cheekbones with your fingertips. Roll baby over and rub from the feet up the backs of the legs. Finally, massage baby's back using long, gentle strokes. End, if your baby allows you, with a gentle sacral rock. With your baby still lying on their tummy, place one palm on the small of baby's lower back and the other palm in the upper middle of the back. Gently rock the baby from side to side, moving only the hand at the lower back. Keep your upper hand still. You will notice that the baby has their own rhythm. Try to tune in to the child's speed, not your own. Gently rock to your baby's own tune. This will help the child prepare for sleep. Do this for as long as baby will allow.

If you want to try some sleepytime massage on your older children, begin by placing both of your hands on your child's back on either side of the spine, and move your palms up, out, back down, and around to make little heart shapes. Move your hands in a slow, steady rhythm, and let the love you feel for your child flow through your hands and into their body. Another move you can use is the figure eight. Using the pads of your fingertips, very gently trace a large figure eight on your child's back. Think of the energy within the child's body flowing smoothly with a positive vibration as you trace the figure.

Restful Sleep Charm

To encourage your baby or older child to sleep soundly throughout the night, try this charm, which doubles as a general blessing for love and protection. Choose a piece of lavender or purple paper, and in the middle of it, write the following (for older children, simply substitute the word "baby" with "child"):

By the light of the moon in the black sky above,
My baby will slumber wrapped up in my love!
By the light of the sun when it comes up again,
My baby will give me a good morning grin!

In the left-hand margin to the left of these words, draw the moon. For best effect, depict it as a full moon or waxing crescent. Beneath the moon, draw a clock showing the time that represents your idea of an ideal bedtime for your child. In the right-hand margin to the right of the words, draw the sun. Beneath it, draw a clock showing the time at which you want your baby or child to wake up.

Next, take the paper outside at night after the moon has risen. Spend some time enjoying the nighttime; do a little stargazing if possible. Let the moonlight wash over the paper, filling it with a soothing, dreamy vibration. Read the first line of the verse you wrote on the paper (the "By the light of the moon..." part). Close your eyes and feel your motherly love well up in your heart. Imagine that love as a warm, soft blanket wrapped gently around your child. Take some slow, deep breaths as if you were dozing, and as you do so, visualize your child sleeping soundly through-out the night. See in your mind's eye a clock depicting bedtime, and imag-ine the hands of the clock moving around and around slowly through all the hours of the night. Open your eyes and end the visualization just be-fore the clock's hands reach the morning wake-up time. Leave the paper outside overnight, taking care to weigh it down with something and also keeping it away from direct contact with the dewy grass.

In the morning after the sun comes up, go outside, retrieve the pa-per, and read the remaining line of the verse (the "By the light of the sun..." part). Let the sunlight stream through the paper, warming it, illuminating it. Visualize that clock again, this time seeing the hands advance just beyond your ideal wake-up time. Imagine your precious wee one waking up with a big, happy grin, eyes filled with a joyful, dancing light. Smile brightly at the paper and take it back inside. If you like, rub some dried or fresh chamomile or lavender over the paper to further strengthen the magick. Your restful sleep charm is now ready for use. Put the paper in an attractive picture frame or hang it up as is, somewhere out of reach near your child's bed.

No More Bad Dreams Sachet

Use this sachet to help encourage happy dreams and keep nightmares at bay. You will need the following:

¼ cup sea salt

¼ cup lavender (fresh or dried flowers and leaves)

A few drops of spring water or holy water

Hold the sea salt in your hands and think of the fear and anxiety your child is experiencing due to bad dreams. Think of the shadowy dark-ness, the uncertainty of the unknown. Touch the salt with your finger-tips and envision these fears being absorbed into the salt, eaten up and neutralized by the salt's purifying qualities. Say out loud or to yourself, "This salt absorbs the darkness and the shadows that dwell therein! This salt will purify! This salt will cleanse!"

Now mix the lavender into the salt. Think of your child sleeping peacefully, happily. Let yourself daydream and imagine in detail the whimsical, happy dreams you would like your child to enjoy. Go there in your mind; experience the sights, sounds, and pleasures of this happy dream scene. Imagine your child's slumbering, smiling face, and let the joyful and loving feelings well up in your heart. Feel the peace of that love, and envision that loving, happy energy surrounding your child in an orb glowing with lavender light. Say out loud or to yourself, "This lavender brings love! This lavender brings joy! This lavender brings happy dreams!"

Continue to mix the lavender and salt together with your fingertips. Let their energies blend together, the peace and joy of the lavender combining with the purity and protection supplied by the salt. Finally, sprinkle in a few drops of the water. Think of the divine energies of the water entering the lavender and salt to further empower and bind those energies together. Wrap the mixture up in a white or lavender-colored cloth; twist it up and secure the top with white or red thread to create a little bundle, or sachet. Hold the sachet in your hands and say emphatically while envisioning your child sleeping contentedly, "Good dreams! Happy dreams! Bad dreams are no more! Good dreams! Happy dreams! Only good dreams forever more!"

Place the sachet under a pillow or under the bed, or tie it to the bedpost if your child is old enough. For children three and under, place the sachet somewhere in the bedroom but well out of reach so that it doesn't present a choking danger or become a midnight snack.

The Restful Ruse

This trick is pretty crafty, but it's often successful when all else has failed. If your child is stubbornly refusing to sleep and insisting that you stay in the room with them, sit quietly and after a couple of minutes close your eyes. Slow your breathing to a sleeping pace, and do your best to pretend like you have dozed off. Once the little one realizes Mommy has fallen asleep, they're likely to quickly follow suit. The hard part is making sure you don't actually fall asleep for real while trying to fool your kiddo.

Blanket of Love Charm

Use this charm to help your child feel safe and cared for throughout the night. Simply hold the child's blanket or other bedding close to your heart and hug it as you think about how much you love your child. Imagine yourself cuddling and comforting your child. Feel your heart expand with love and joy, and put all those warm and fuzzy feelings into the blanket. Your little one will feel the comfort of your arms as they drift off to sleep with their enchanted blanket.

Making the Most of Bedtime

Bedtime is a magickal time when everyday reality is left behind and our subconscious minds are allowed to soar unencumbered by the physical body. Watching your baby or child sleeping peacefully is one of the most precious sights a mother can experience. If you're too set on your expectations being met, however, bedtime can become very stressful. Try to let go of your own anxiety, and even if you're not feeling calm, fake it as best you can. The more relaxed you are, the more relaxed your child will be, too. No matter how bad it gets, keep in mind that your child will eventually fall asleep, so take heart—you're almost off duty. With a serene aura surrounding you and the tips and tricks in this chapter in hand, bedtime can be a pleasant and special highlight of the day.

Chapter 13

Mealtime Magick

Around the world, cultural, religious, and spiritual beliefs regarding the energetic properties and magick of food abound. In the Hindu yogic tradition, foods are divided into three categories according to basic energetic quality and effect on the body: *tamasic* foods, such as mushrooms, meat, and alcohol, which dull the mind; *rajasic* foods, such as garlic, onions, and other spicy or salty foods, which excite the mind; and *sattvic* foods, which support good health and mental clarity.

Foods that are grown naturally and are minimally processed are believed to be more sattvic and contain more *prana* (life force energy) than foods that are grown with chemicals or are heavily processed. Prana is the energy that keeps us healthy, energized, spiritually attuned, and emotionally balanced. All foods contain some measure of prana, but you'll find more of it in sattvic foods (such as naturally produced dairy products and organically grown fresh fruits, grains, cereals, legumes, nuts, and veggies) than you'll find in meat or in overly processed or overly spicy food products. Sattvic foods are considered the most pure. These foods often have a sweet taste, and babies, as pure as any human being will ever be, naturally crave sweet tastes over any other flavor. Among the most sattvic and prana-rich foods are mango, banana, apple, pear, and sweet potato—which, incidentally, all make excellent first foods for baby. For good health and optimal energy, incorporate sattvic foods often into your family's balanced diet.

Of course, choosing the best foods to prepare is just one part of the equation for making mealtimes more magickal. There are many other ways to enhance the energy and bring out the magickal properties of your food. In this chapter, you'll learn some techniques for magickal food preparation and cooking, and you'll also discover some tips for preparing easy, all-natural, and affordable baby food.

Enhancing the Magick of Food

To bring out the prana in your food and awaken its unique magickal attributes, hold your hands on or over the food and try to sense the energies moving through it. Can you sense a pulsing, a vibration? This is the prana, the energy. Focus on this energy, and envision it magnifying, growing brighter and bigger and bolder. If you're aware of any particular attribute of the food—such as apples being good for encouraging happiness, for instance—think of that attribute now and express your intention for the food to reveal and emphasize this aspect of itself. Send as much good, loving, happy energy into the food as you can. If you like, say a simple blessing over the food, something in your own words that speaks to your personal beliefs.

Food Prep with Magick in Mind

In addition to activating and enhancing the prana of your food, you can also use various food preparation techniques as an opportunity to make your meals more magickal. As you work with ingredients, think about the energies that you want to bring out in the food and the intention of the meal. While the main purpose of the meal is to nourish the body, it can also nourish the mind and soul as well. Cook with love, joy, and peace in your heart, and try incorporating the following magickal food preparation techniques.

Peeling: Whenever you peel fruit or vegetables, you can perform
a little sympathetic magick for stress reduction. Hold the fruit
or vegetable in your hands and think about who will eat this food.

Think about the stress, anxiety, or frustration that this person may experience. As you peel the vegetable, imagine that you are also peeling away these negative feelings, lessening the stress, removing the frustration as each strip of peel comes loose.

Slicing: Cutting up ingredients offers another chance to incorporate a little magick into your day. Hold the knife and think about the quality you wish to impart to the food you're slicing, be it happiness, love, peace, or another feeling. Conjure up this emotion as strongly as you can; imagine that you are filled to the brim with the desired quality. Send this feeling down your arm, out through your hand, and into the knife's handle and blade. As you chop, slice, and dice, the knife will impart its magickal energies to the food.

Boiling: Boiling is another effective medium for kitchen magick. As the water heats, whatever energetic qualities that water has are magnified and infused into the food that cooks within it. Water is very versatile and neutral in nature, like a blank slate that you can enchant with whatever properties you wish. When enchanting water to use for cooking, choose a positive energy such as joy, laughter, relaxation, unity, or cooperation. Think of this energy as you fill the pot with water. Tell the water what to do; instruct it to carry out your intentions. As the water comes to a boil, think about the energies within that water becoming amplified, the water's power growing exponentially as the bubbles break the surface. Place the food in the pot, and as it boils, envision the energies of the water seeping into the food, enchanting it with the same magickal properties.

Mashing: If you've got a baby in the house, chances are you have ample occasions for mashing up various foods. Luckily, you can make this tedious chore into an act of magick that will help dissolve obstacles and achieve breakthroughs. Has your child been presenting any special challenges lately, such as being especially cranky, or not sleeping well, or engaging in an unwanted habit? As you mash up the food, imagine that you are mashing up these obstacles, smashing through any barriers to a happier and more peaceful existence.

Stirring: The next time you're mixing up baby food or a big pot of stew, why not stir up some magick while you're at it? Start by enchanting the spoon you'll be using. Hold the utensil and think about your magickal intention, imagining the outcome you desire as clearly and as vividly as possible. Do you want the food to be healing, energizing, or calming? Do you want the food to foster good feelings between the members of your family? Think about your intention as you hold the spoon, and envision those thoughts flowing into it, charging it up with your will. As you stir the food, visualize the energies in the spoon radiating outward into the food, aligning the ingredients with your intention. You can also draw symbols in the food as you stir, using the spoon to trace a heart for love, a star for power or protection, or a four-leaf clover for luck or happiness.

Making Baby Food

While those little ready-packed jars of baby food are certainly cute and convenient, it's much more cost-effective, healthy, and fun to make your own baby food at home. Making your own baby food gives you the most control over the end product, especially if you are a magickal mom who wants to infuse your baby's foods with as much love and intention as possible. Here are just a few of the benefits of making your own baby food:

- You know exactly what's in it.
- There are no fillers and no chemicals needed to keep it fresh. Your freezer will do just fine.
- You can infuse the food with whatever magickal intentions you like, right from the very start of the cooking process.
- You can mix and match various fruits and veggies as you see fit, creating your own unique combinations for your baby.

The main reason mothers opt out of making their own baby food is convenience. The perception that baby-food making is time-consuming or difficult is common but misguided. By implementing just a couple of simple strategies, your homemade baby food will be every bit as convenient as the store-bought stuff. The first strategy is to make the food in bulk. Make a big batch once a week, then store the food in ice cube trays.

While a good rule of thumb is to start baby on solid foods only after they can sit upright on their own without support, always follow your doctor's recommendations. When you first start your baby on solids, feed them only one food at a time for a few days up to a week before moving on to a new food. This way, you'll be able to immediately spot and identify any allergic reactions to the food your baby might have, and you won't have to do an elimination process to figure out which particular ingredient is the culprit.

At the beginning, your baby will eat primarily as a way to practice chewing, develop their sense of taste, and prepare themselves for culinary adventures to come. If you're nursing, starting your baby on solids when the time is right will also give you a little break so you're not so constantly in demand for feedings. At this stage, vegetable and fruit purees make a nice addition to iron-fortified, single-grain baby cereals. You might try your baby on sweet potatoes, carrots, pears, prunes, avocados, bananas, peaches, or other fruits and vegetables. Puree the food to a smooth, runny consistency to start, and as your baby cuts teeth and develops their chewing abilities, switch from purees to mashed ingredients.

Making your own vegetable and fruit purees and mashes is easy. Here's what you'll need:

Steamer basket
Vegetable peeler
Ice cube trays
Cutting board
Sharp knife
Large pan, pot, or Dutch oven (filled with water)
Blender
Gallon-sized plastic food storage bags or freezer bags
Storage containers for on-the-go daily activities

Start by peeling your fruit or vegetable, then chop it into medium-sized chunks. Place the steamer basket over a pan, pot, or Dutch oven filled with water to a point just under the basket. You don't want the water to seep up through the bottom of the steamer basket, so keep the water level just beneath it. Bring the water to a boil, place the food in the steamer basket, cover, and cook until soft enough to easily mash with a fork. If you don't have a steamer basket, simply boil the vegetables or fruit in roughly one inch of water—just enough to cover them. Let the water come to a boil first before adding the food, and check the water level periodically throughout the cooking process.

Cooking time will vary based on the size and density of the fruit or vegetable and whether you are steaming or boiling. Steaming takes longer, but it allows the food to retain more nutrients. For softer foods like apples, pears, mangoes, broccoli, or cauliflower, check for tenderness after about fifteen to twenty minutes if you're steaming and after about ten to fifteen minutes if you're boiling. Sweet potatoes, squash, and carrots take longer; allow about thirty minutes or more if you're steaming and about twenty-five minutes if you're boiling. You want to cook the fruits and veggies longer than you would for an adult so that the food is easy to mash or puree and will not present a choking hazard for baby. Once the food starts to soften, check it every few minutes until it's ready. The food will be very hot, so use a mitten to pull the steamer basket up, carefully letting any excess water drain out through the bottom of the basket. If you boiled your ingredients, strain them in a colander. Let the food cool thoroughly.

Next, it's time to get the food baby-ready. If you're going for a puree, put the food in the blender and use the puree or liquefy setting until it's smooth and chunk-free and about the same consistency as yogurt or mashed potatoes. If you're making food for an older baby who is ready and able to chew up chunkier foods, simply mash the fruits or vegetables using the back of a fork. Go for a mixed consistency, mashing some of it very thoroughly and leaving a few half-mashed pieces here and there. Just make sure you don't leave behind any solid chunks large enough to present a choking risk. If you'd like to make the fruits or vegetables a little creamier, try adding a splash of water, coconut water, or pumped breast milk. The breast milk helps make the food easier to digest for a baby who is just beginning this culinary experience, while the coconut water adds extra flavor and nutrition. About ¼ cup of liquid per every two to three cups of baby food will do.

Put some of the fresh food into a storage container to keep in the fridge. Glass containers are best, as they help protect the energy and magick of the food, but any BPA-free, airtight container will do. Cooked fruits and veggies stored in the fridge should be used within forty-eight hours, so put away just enough to last your baby through two days of feedings. Pour the remainder of the food into ice cube trays, then cover with plastic wrap and place them in the freezer. Frozen baby food can last as long as three to six months, but try to use it within a month or two for freshest taste. Once the food has frozen, transfer the cubes into freezer bags for more convenient storage. Putting the cubes into bags also allows you to mix and match the cubes to create bags of your baby's favorites. For instance, one bag might contain a variety of fruit cubes that taste good together, and another a variety of vegetable cubes that combine well. Be sure to label the bags with both contents and date.

The frozen cubes can be thawed out overnight in the refrigerator; just pull them out fifteen to thirty minutes before serving so the food can come to room temperature. Microwaving baby food is risky, as it can create hot spots in the food that could hurt baby. If you're careful to stir the food thoroughly and check it for temperature consistency, however, microwaving is an effective option. Just put the cubes in a glass bowl and heat in fifteen-second increments at medium power until melted, stirring after each interval. Allow the food to cool completely and stir it well before serving.

The baby food can also be thawed out on the stove top; just place it in a skillet and heat over medium-low heat until thoroughly melted. As with the microwave heating method, be sure to let the food cool back to room temperature before serving, and stir thoroughly. Another way to thaw frozen baby food cubes is to place them in a bowl (or leave them in the freezer bag) and submerge this in a larger container of hot water. This method will take around fifteen to twenty minutes. If you've opted to thaw the cubes right in the bag, you may need to weigh it down with a heavy cup or saucer to keep it under the water. If you're going to be out and about all day, simply take the frozen cubes with you in an insulated lunch bag or cooler along with an ice pack, and thaw when needed. You can find handy one- to two-ounce storage containers that will hold about one cube of food each. These make on-the-go baby feeding a breeze, as you can use the container as a bowl and don't have to carry any additional dishes.

First Foods for Babies and Their Magickal Attributes

Here is a sampling of foods most commonly given to babies who are beginning to eat solids, along with a description of each food's magickal attributes and energetic qualities. Always choose foods with nutrition in mind first, then bring out the magick of the food you've selected by envisioning its particular qualities charging the dish with energy and loving intention.

Apple: Love, happiness, healing, peace, beauty, vitality.

Avocado: Beauty, love, calming, dreams.

Banana: Calming, contentment, intelligence, prosperity.

Broccoli: Health, protection, strength, abundance.

Carrot: Luck, power, energy, insight, clear vision.

Cauliflower: Relaxation, stamina, peace, healing.

Mango: Cheerfulness, satisfaction, love, luck.

Pear: Longevity, blessings, comfort, solitude.

Sweet Potato: Health, strength, growth, prosperity.

Yummy Food Mixes for Baby

Once your baby has some experience eating, they'll probably be ready to experiment with different combinations of their favorite foods. Remember to try baby on each ingredient individually to start, and only move on to mixed foods once you're certain your child can tolerate every component. Always follow your doctor's recommendations about what to feed baby and when to start.

Here are a few yummy food mixes to try for baby. We've left out the use of any berries, melons, or citrus fruits in our recipes, as these foods tend to be more allergenic.

- Pear, apple, and sweet potato. You can use any or all of these ingredients to help thicken or sweeten any other baby-food blend you might make. They also taste great together on their own.
- Avocado and banana. This combination is delicious and packed full of essential fatty acids, powerful nutrients, and positive energy.
- Avocado, banana, pear, and coconut water. This mixture is so sweet and yummy that it could be a dessert, yet it's very nutritious.
- Sweet potato, carrot, butternut squash, and apple. This combination is hearty and filling yet sweet enough to gain your baby's approval. You can substitute pear or mango for the apple.
- Sweet potato and cauliflower. This blend will help your baby get used to more savory flavors while incorporating a light touch of sweetness from the potato. Try mixing this with baby cereal.

Picky Eaters and How to Deal

As your little one gets older and more choosy, you may have to get more creative in your food choices. Toddlers naturally become much more picky. It's part of the deal of becoming a toddler. They are discovering who they are and what they like, and they want you to know their personality and preferences. Just try to be reasonably flexible and keep in mind that you can always sneak in healthy ingredients. You may have to do pre-packaged organic oatmeal instead of the somewhat healthier non-pre-packaged variety if that's the only thing your toddler will eat, for instance, but you can always add in flaxseed meal, ground-up almonds or walnuts, chia seeds, hemp seeds, and organic raisins to up the nutrient profile.

For snacks, try Greek yogurt mixed with powdered ranch dressing to serve as a healthy dip for veggies or veggie chips. Parsnips are a good choice for a palatable veggie that can be mixed in with other foods. Try adding veggies to a "pizza" made with a flour tortilla that's coated with a very small amount of spaghetti sauce, sprinkled with cheese, and baked in the oven for a few minutes. Smoothies are another tasty way to work more nutrient-rich foods into your picky eater's diet; just blend yogurt with fresh or frozen fruit, flax, or other healthy ingredients. Tuck some black beans into a quesadilla for added protein. Pick your battles, and sneak in healthy additions wherever you can.

Another good way to encourage kids to eat well is to get them involved in the food preparation. As your baby grows into a toddler and then into a full-fledged kid, allow them to take a greater role in your family's meal planning. Let them pick out which new fruit or vegetable they want to try next, or let them choose a healthy snack for the family.

Your child will likely go through many eating phases, first adamantly refusing a food and then later devouring it, or deciding that the only thing worth eating in the world is goldfish crackers. It's your job as a parent to ensure your child is getting adequate nutrition, but as long as that's taken care of, you have room to be flexible and make adjustments as your child's dietary needs and tastes change. Don't give up too easily on any one food; simply try it again later, as persistence can often pay off. Getting your kids to eat healthy often becomes more of a challenge as they grow up, but if you're creative and determined, you can make it happen.

Chapter 14

~~ ᦅ·ᦕ ~~

Magickal Home

As mothers, we're likely to spend a good portion of each day in the home. Even if you work outside the house, there's still cleaning to do, meals to prepare and consume, sleeping to do, guests to host, and family fun to be had all within the confines of home. If your home is messy, cluttered, and filled with stale, negative energies, it will start to feel like a prison fast. By adding in some magickal touches and incorporating good feng shui, your home will feel like a nurturing sanctuary in no time. In this chapter, you'll learn some ways to keep your home feeling safe, blessed, protected, and filled with positive vibrations. The home truly is the heart of the family, so make yours the best it can be.

Crystals and Stones

Crystals and stones provide a great way to add positive energy to your home. Each stone or crystal has its own special properties that can be utilized in a variety of ways, from deflecting negativity to encouraging good cheer. If you have babies or small children in the home, be sure to keep stones up high out of reach, and if possible choose larger sizes that are too big to fit in the mouth.

Keep your crystals and stones clean. While typically your stones and crystals will retain their positive energy as long as they're not exposed to bad energies, it's a good idea to clean them every few months just in case, to clear them of any ickiness they may have picked up. You may want to cleanse them monthly on each full moon. To purify and recharge your rocks, simply rub them with salt, rinse them with water, or place them beneath the sunlight or moonlight for a few hours. Here are a few easy ways to use crystals and stones to improve your home's energy.

To Absorb and Neutralize Negativity

If there is anger or depression in your home and you'd like to dispel it, try placing several large hunks of jet around the house. This black stone will siphon the negative energies away from the home's inhabitants. It can also be used to help ward off bad dreams.

To Bring Peace and Harmony

To create an all-around peaceful, pleasant vibe that will help the people in your home feel good toward one another and get along well together, try placing pieces of rose quartz and/or turquoise around your dwelling.

To Increase Cheerfulness

If you want to cultivate a more cheerful, happy, upbeat atmosphere, try placing citrine crystals or clear quartz crystals around your home to help lift the general vibe.

For Healing and Purifying

To help balance and restore your body's energies while you sleep, place an arrangement of stones beneath your bed, choosing large specimens that don't present a choking hazard. You might arrange the stones beneath the bed so that they correspond to your body's chakras. Place a hematite near the foot of your bed to correspond to the energy center located at your feet, and above that place a red or orange calcite to correspond with the chakra located at your pelvis. A yellow calcite comes next to correspond with the chakra located at the solar plexus, and a fluorite or green calcite is placed to correspond with the energy centered at the heart. Next, place a blue celestite to align with your throat chakra, and an amethyst to align with the third eye chakra located between your eyes. Finally, place a clear quartz to correspond with the crown chakra located at the very top of the head. This arrangement will help replenish and balance your body's natural strength and vigor. You can substitute these stones with any others of the same color or similar vibration. Let your intuition guide your selections.

Plants

Living plants add oxygen and positive, vital energy to the home, and they can also provide clues about the general well-being of your household. When plants are thriving, it's a good confirmation that your family is likely thriving, too. If your plants suddenly wilt or become diseased, however, it can be a warning that you may be neglecting other things in your life in addition to the plant-care duties. If your plants are struggling, give them love and attention and all the light and water they need to grow. Give these things also to your loved ones, nurturing them with love, attention, food, and drink.

There are many indoor and outdoor plants to choose from. With kids or animals in the house, it's best to stick with non-poisonous plants only. Place the plants in hanging baskets or on high shelves out of the reach of babies, toddlers, and pets who might otherwise be tempted to dig in the dirt or tear and eat the leaves. If you like to cook, you might consider growing culinary herbs in a row of small pots placed on a wall shelf in the kitchen. Consider growing versatile herbs such as rosemary, basil, and oregano that can be used for cooking and magick alike. You might hang a pot of lavender in your living room to help mellow the vibe, or place a pot of daisies on your dining table to encourage friendship and good feelings while your family dines. You don't have to overload your house with plants. Just add enough here and there so that some of that beautiful plant energy and fresh oxygen can enter your home.

Bagua Mirrors

A bagua is a small, round mirror typically set into a wooden, octagonal frame. Bagua mirrors are usually around four to six inches in diameter, but can be much larger. The frame of the bagua is divided into sections and decorated with trigrams to represent the harmonious flow of energy throughout different aspects of your life, from career to love to family. These mirrors are said to reflect and return any energy that is not of the highest vibration.

Bagua mirrors can be hung outside the house over main entrances or anyplace else where you feel like negative energy is entering your home. If you live in a dangerous neighborhood or have very unfriendly neighbors, you might consider placing a bagua mirror on each exterior wall of your home so that negative energies will be deflected regardless of which direction they come from. Many feng shui experts advise against using a bagua inside the home, as the negative energy it deflects would merely be bounced back into the enclosed space. Intention rules, though, so if you feel inclined to try a bagua indoors, just be sure to place a piece of jet stone, a bundle of sage or rosemary, a dried lemon, or another energy-absorbing and neutralizing object somewhere nearby to act as the collection point for all the icky vibrations reflected by the mirror.

Magickal Scents for the Home

Scent offers another medium through which to add energy and harmonize the vibrations of your home. You might use scents in the form of potpourri, room spray, scented cleaners, scented hand soaps, sachets, scented candles, diffusers, or oil burners. You might even create your own makeshift simmer pot, placing fruit rinds or spices in a small amount of water in a saucepan that's heated on the stove over low to medium heat.

Just be sure to use scents safely, given the inhabitants of your home. If anyone has asthma or other breathing difficulties, avoid artificial scents, aerosol sprays, and strong odors of any kind. With babies, small children, or pets around, use scent sparingly, be sure to investigate any herbs or essential oils you're using to make sure they're not toxic, and try to avoid the use of harsh chemical sprays. Place potpourri or other loose herbs up high and out of reach. You can wrap loose herbs in cloth, tie the top, and create a sachet that can be hung securely from the ceiling to freshen the air. For a stronger scent, sprinkle the herbs with essential oil. Try the following scents for different effects.

Apple: Use to boost feelings of love, happiness, and friendship.

Cinnamon: Use to increase energy, boost enthusiasm, and fuel passions.

Citrus: Use to encourage cheerfulness or increase energy, or to refresh, rejuvenate, and purify.

Floral: Use to encourage peace and love, bring inspiration, and enhance beauty.

Vanilla: Use to encourage passion, love, and warmth, or to bring comfort or enhance psychic abilities.

Pentacle of Protection Charm

Here is a simple charm you can use to help improve the general energy and atmosphere of your home. With a stick of incense, a bundle of sage, or a quartz crystal in your hand, face the north. Use the incense, sage, or crystal to trace the outline of a pentacle. As you do so, think of the strong, protective earth guarding your home. Envision the strength of a thousand mountains standing behind you. Now turn to the east, imagining powerful winds blowing through your home and clearing out any stale, unwanted energies. Now turn to the south, envisioning the heat, strength, and brightness of the sun that illuminates all shadows and eliminates all darkness; imagine this light shining brilliantly within your home. Finally, turn to the west, feeling the insistence and grace of the ocean tides washing away distress and bringing good energies into your home. Trace the pentacle as you face each direction in turn. You can do this once in the main area of your house, or go room by room and perform the whole circuit of the four directions in each room. Do whatever time allows or whatever you feel is needed. This simple charm will bless your home with power and protection.

Threshold Shield for Protection

To guard your home from unwanted individuals and to keep negative energies out, craft this simple charm and place it under the doormat outside your home. Take a piece of ordinary paper and, beginning on the outside edge, write the following words in a spiral that curves around and around inwardly toward the center of the paper:

Intruders, thieves, evil entities! Anger, shame, greed, and jealousy!
You cannot pass! You go in here! You cannot cross this threshold here!
You go in here and you are trapped! You can't get out! You cannot pass!

When you get to the end of the words, draw a big X right in the middle of the page. Replace the charm annually, or sooner if you feel your home has had to fend off any major threats. When you install a fresh charm, burn or shred the old one.

Threshold Blessing Charm

Use this charm to invite good energies into your home. First, choose a sprig of fresh herbs, a flower, or a crystal that you feel has the type of energies that you want to welcome into your living space. For instance, you might choose a sprig of rosemary to welcome in love and positive energy. You might select a daisy to represent friendship, or a sprig of pine, oregano, or basil to represent wealth. Perhaps a citrine crystal best represents the good cheer and happiness you wish to invite into your home. Trust your intuition and choose something that calls to you.

Whatever you choose, hold it in your hand and stand with it outside your front door. Feel its vibration, and think about the positive energies that are welcome to cross your threshold. Move the herb or stone or whatever you've chosen in wide concentric circles in front of the door, envisioning the desired energies rushing into your home, blessing it and enchanting it so that the house itself attracts and invites in whatever it is you seek. Wrap the herb or stone (or whatever else you used) in white cloth, bind it with red thread, and hang it securely above the door.

Elemental Power and Protection Ritual

Here's a simple ritual you can use to purify and enchant your home with the power and protection of the four elements: earth, air, water, and fire. First, clean the room in which you will be performing the ritual. You might perform the ritual in each room of your house, or simply perform it in a main area such as the living room or near the front door. Declutter the space, dust off any surfaces that need to be wiped down, and remove any garbage. The room doesn't have to be entirely spotless. Just do something to spruce it up a bit, and clean as much as you feel you need to.

In each corner of the room, place a symbol of each of the four elements. Use incense, a feather, or a fan for the air element; a glass bowl or cup of water for the water element; a dish of salt or soil to represent the earth element; and a lit candle to represent the element of fire. You can place these elemental symbols randomly, one in each corner, or you can assign them according to the cardinal directions, placing the symbol of earth to the north, the symbol of air to the east, the symbol of fire to the south, and the symbol of water to the west. If there are any babies, pets, or small children in the house, you'll have to get them out of the area while you do this ritual, or else place the items up high and out of reach.

When you're ready to place the symbols of the elements in each corner, think of the energies and properties that are being represented here in your space. As you place the incense, feather, or fan, think about how the air element creates movement. It is the breath. It is the cool breeze that carries the seeds and clears the clouds. As you place the water, think of how this element quenches thirst and sustains life. Envision a flowing river cutting a path through a solid rock wall, and think of how water transforms everything it touches. As you place the soil or salt, think of how the earth element provides us with a solid foundation, a strong, stable force on which we can rely. As you place the candle, think of the fiery sun warming the earth. Think of a wall of flames turning a pile of obstacles into ashes. Think of the light from a campfire illuminating the surrounding ground.

Ask each of the four elements in turn to enter your space, to bless it and protect it. Finally, sprinkle a small pinch of sea salt in each corner of the room to help further absorb and purify any lingering negative energies. You'll be amazed at how quickly this little ritual can completely transform a room's energy, leaving the space feeling cleansed, protected, and empowered.

Feng Shui for the Nursery

"A baby's nursery is very important to their well-being, so we want to make sure they have the best feng shui possible from the moment they arrive home from the hospital," says feng shui consultant Jill Kostrinsky. "A nursery with good feng shui equals a healthy baby, and a good night's sleep for the whole family," she explains. Feng shui is a complex art in which item placement, direction, color, and open space are considered to design rooms with an optimally harmonious and balanced energy flow. There's a lot to it, but luckily you don't have to learn all there is to know in order to reap some of the benefits of feng shui. Try incorporating these simple ideas into the design of your baby's room, and see if you notice your baby becoming happier and calmer as a result:

- If possible, locate the baby's room in the east of the house, as feng shui teaches that this is the area corresponding to growth and new beginnings.

- Wood works wonders. As Kostrinsky explains, "Babies are quickly growing outward in all directions from center—physically, mentally, and spiritually—so they are considered 'wood' elements in feng shui. In order to support this kind of growth, include some wood energy in their environment." There are many ways to represent the wood element beyond the obvious use of actual wood. Virtually anything tall, rectangular, or columnar could be used to represent this element. In addition to wooden furniture, you might include paintings of trees, straw mats, natural fiber bedding, vertical stripes, or other embellishments to represent the wood element.

- Consider green. With its nurturing, vital vibration, green is a wonderful shade for growing children. Try pale green on walls or bedding to create a serene atmosphere, and incorporate accents of dark green or jewel green here and there to represent your child's bountiful growth and development.

- Keep electronics away from the crib. Baby monitors, clocks, radios, televisions, and other devices can emit electromagnetic fields that can interrupt what might otherwise be a restful night's sleep. Be sure to place such items at least six feet away from the bed.

- Place the crib in a diagonal path to the door. You don't want it to be directly in line with the door, as this is the opening through which energy pours into the room. Locating the crib well out of this main energetic pathway will help your baby's room feel more calm and peaceful. Also, arrange the crib so the head of it (rather than the whole side of it) is against the wall. This will help your baby feel freer and less confined, and will help your child have an unencumbered energy flow. With thoughtful bed placement, the current of energy swirling in through the door will have time and space to slow down before it reaches your wee one.

- Avoid metal furnishings. Metal conducts a lot of energy, which can leave babies feeling overwhelmed and overstimulated. Choose wood, wicker, or fabric designs instead to create a more restful vibe.

Feng Shui for the Adult's Bedroom

You want your bedroom to be a sanctuary of love, a romantic place for you and your partner to be intimate and passionate. If your bedroom is cluttered, dingy, dark, or dismal, it's probably not the sort of environment that puts you in the mood, exactly. On the other hand, with the right atmosphere, romance flows more easily and loving encounters come more naturally. If you're on your own and looking for a partner, making your bedroom more romantic can help draw new love into your life. Of course, the bedroom isn't just a place for romance; you'll want to do at least a little sleeping here as well. Try the following tips for balancing and improving your bedroom feng shui:

- Give special consideration to the placement of your bed. You want the bed to be easily accessible from both sides, and ideally you want to be able to see the door from your bed, but you don't want the bed to be in direct line with the door. Just do the best you can given your bedroom's architectural design and space limitations. Keep the area around and under your bed clean, and make sure you don't have any sharp corners or heavy objects pointing toward the bed.

- Strive for versatile lighting. Bright, natural light works for the day-time, and soft lighting from adjustable lamps or candlelight is per-fect for the evening and night.

- Avoid placing major electronics such as computers or televisions in your bedroom. If you must have these items in your room, consid-er placing them in a cabinet with closed doors or concealing them beneath a cloth or curtain. The energy emitted by such electronics can sow disharmony and disrupt your sleep.

- Also avoid water features such as aquariums or tabletop meditation fountains. Too much water in the bedroom can lead to decreased passion.

- Use natural earth tones such as whites, tans, browns, oranges, pinks, and corals to create a pleasant, comfortable atmosphere in the bed-room. You can use splashes of fiery colors like bright red to help turn up the heat, but be aware that an overabundance of hot and vibrant hues can interfere with rest and increase irritability. Darker reds that have a more earthy feel, however, can be used more liberally.

- Lean toward a minimalist approach and choose wisely what you keep in your bedroom. Don't let it become a storage area for clut-ter. Clutter includes an overabundance of shoes and/or books; do your best to store these items in another area of your home. Value the open space, and keep only what you absolutely want or need in your bedroom.

- Select a few romance-inspiring items, be they sentimental photos, art prints of romantic places, or statues of beautiful, lusty god-desses. You don't want to overdo it, but a smattering of objects especially chosen to inspire the passions or stir up fond memories can go far in fostering feelings of romance and intimacy.

- Use lust-inspiring scents such as jasmine, ylang-ylang, rose, sandal-wood, vanilla, or patchouli in the bedroom.

- Hang a crystal or glass orb near the doorway of your bedroom to improve the general energy flow.

- Incorporate subtle flower imagery in your bedroom to create a romantic vibe.

- Include in your bedroom décor a pair of items to symbolize love and togetherness, such as a set of similar figurines or a pair of matching candlesticks.

- Place love-attracting, passion-boosting crystals, stones, or metals such as rose quartz, amethyst, aquamarine, jade, copper, or silver in the bedroom.

- Incorporate love symbols into the room. Consider dragon and phoenix imagery, or figurines or paintings of birds, lotuses, fish, or elephants.

- To encourage more passion and lust in the bedroom, invite in the fire element. Hang a red paper lantern or place a small lamp with a red shade near the bed. Red candles are also effective. Just be sure you don't fall asleep with candles burning.

- Avoid having reminders of non-romantic familial life in your bedroom. This is a relaxing space for you and your partner, or for yourself and perhaps a future partner, if you are on your own. Do your best to keep your bedroom free of items that will remind you of all the millions of other things you need to do besides relaxing and all the countless obligations you must meet in order to care for the people who rely on you. This means no stacks of diapers, no stacks of work, no piles of bills, no dirty laundry, and no pictures of children, parents, or other relatives.

The Magickal Kitchen

Whether or not you're the cook of your household, you'll likely spend enough time in the kitchen to warrant sprucing it up a little. Here are some quick tips to make your kitchen space sing:

- Use bright colors and earth tones to create a cheerful, harmonious, nurturing vibe in the kitchen. Keep color symbolism in mind if you like, using yellows to represent sunshine and happiness; greens for nurturing, growth, health, and prosperity; whites for purity; and browns for strength and stability.

- Place potted plants in your kitchen to attract good luck. For further benefits, grow versatile kitchen herbs such as basil, oregano, and rosemary that can be used for both culinary and magickal purposes.

- Keep the kitchen clean and clutter-free. It's a challenge to do so, but as the heart of the home, the kitchen insists on receiving adequate care and respect. A clean kitchen helps encourage family harmony, whereas a dirty kitchen creates an atmosphere that attracts arguments and negativity.

- Hang a broom in your kitchen as a charm for protection against fire and for blessings upon the family and the food.

- Hang a string of garlic in your kitchen to help absorb negative energies.

- Use citrus scents in your kitchen to create a happy, uplifting atmosphere reminiscent of sunshine. To invite powerful solar energies for success or cheerfulness into your kitchen, boil a pot of water on the stove and add to it one orange, unpeeled but cut into pieces, and a teaspoon or two of cinnamon. As the fragrance fills the air, think of the sun's strength, power, and luminescence enchanting your kitchen to be more conducive to making your magickal wishes manifest.

- Keep your kitchen brightly lit, with plenty of natural light if possible.

- To attract good energies, display fresh fruit in your kitchen and/or hang artwork depicting fruit. Choose grapes to symbolize wealth and health, apples to promote peace and harmony, lemons to purify and energize the general atmosphere, or oranges to attract good luck, success, and prosperity.

- Invite into your kitchen the blessings of Hestia, the Greek goddess of hearth and home, by incorporating some of her symbols into your kitchen décor. Circles, keys, and flames are all sacred to her. You might consider a display of candles, a wreath, or even a bowl of special keys to symbolize the goddess and to ask for her protection.

- Do your best to keep a stock of dried beans and grains in your kitchen to invite abundance and maintain prosperity.

- Place a figurine or other image of a rooster in your kitchen to promote good fortune for the family.

- Avoid plastics whenever possible. Woods and metals have more potent earth energies that are better for the kitchen.

- Place a burnt matchstick or a needle beneath the stove as a magickal deterrent to accidental kitchen fires and to repel negative energies.

Good Energy for the Bathroom

The bathroom is certainly one of the most necessary rooms of the house, so why not give it a little extra love and attention to make it a place of magick? Try these tips to help keep the energies of your bathroom flowing nicely:

- Keep your bathroom clean. A dirty bathroom breeds germs as well as stagnant energies that can leave you feeling down in more ways than one.

- Close the toilet lid and plug drains when not in use. This helps keep the good energy of the space from escaping down the drain.

- Place shells or a small dish or vial of sand in your bathroom to invite in the energies of the ocean. To help increase the potency of the water element within the space, you might add other ocean symbols, such as a mermaid figurine, a ship in a bottle, or a painting of the sea.

- Use cool, clean colors reminiscent of water and nature to help invoke a calming, purifying, revitalizing energy in your bathroom. Whites, greens, and blues make for a harmonious blend.

- Use bright lights or white or yellow candles to invoke solar energies into the room, brightening up the space and enchanting it with the power to recharge and refresh all who enter.

- Include an image of a rayed sun, an eye, or antlers to invoke the healing qualities, protective abilities, and psychic prowess of Sulis, the Roman goddess of hot springs and baths.
- Hang metal wind chimes or bells in your bathroom to help bring balance and to clear out any stale, negative energies.

Magick for the Living Room

Second only to the kitchen, the living room is often one of the top places of congregation in a home. Keeping it even reasonably clean can be a struggle, so make it easier on yourself by planning for a mess. Consider ottomans with hidden storage compartments, lidded baskets, sofas with space underneath, plenty of shelving, and other additions to help stow away the clutter that's bound to accumulate in the living room every time you turn your back. Also, make the space as nice and comfortable as possible. The more magickal you can make your space, the more motivated will you be to take care of it. Here are some tips to bring out the best in your living room:

- Set up a space in your living room to honor your ancestors. This might be a small table, a mantle, a shelf, or a space on the wall. Include photos and other mementos. Place fresh flowers, plants, or candles near the area to help your ancestors feel welcome in your home.
- To cultivate good luck for your family, place a pot of live bamboo in your living room. This will increase joy and attract prosperity.
- For protection and success, include dragon imagery in the living room.
- To attract good fortune and abundance, include a figurine or other image of a cricket in the living room.
- Procure an odd number of Chinese coins, the type with the hole in the middle, and tie these onto a red ribbon, making a total of seven knots. Suspend this from the ceiling on the eastern side of your living room to attract wealth.

- Arrange your couch so it leans against a wall. This provides a feeling of greater comfort and stability than does a "floating" couch placed in the middle of the room and also helps to promote a more harmonious energy flow.

- Avoid placing any furniture with sharp angles directly in line with seating areas, as this creates a negative energy flow that promotes disharmony. Arrange pieces so that corners don't point toward sofas or chairs, and soften hard lines with fabric trim or by placing plants or crystals in or above the area.

- Make sure all family members have a place in the living room. Include items or mementos belonging to each and every person in your household, from the youngest to the oldest, so that everyone feels like a welcomed and included member of the family. This also sends a message to the universe that your family is a united team, a strong pack deserving of respect and good fortune.

- Keep the living room clean and well tended to help promote family happiness, harmony, and cooperation.

- Place a citrine or a clear quartz crystal in your living room to promote happiness, optimism, and good energy. Use a rose quartz to encourage feelings of love and compassion, and a piece of jade to promote good health, success, and longevity.

- Choose relaxing, nurturing earth tones like browns and greens to create a comforting, mellow vibe in your living room.

- To invite balance and increase the general energy and magickal power of the space, include a symbol of each of the four elements in the living room. You might include an aquarium or tabletop fountain to represent water; a candle or lamp for fire; some incense, a fan, a feather, or a picture of the sky for air; and a plant or stone for earth. If you like, arrange these elements to correspond with the cardinal directions: water goes in the west, fire goes in the south, air goes in the east, and earth goes in the north.

The Mom Cave

Every mother deserves her own special area in which to unwind, relax, and steal a few moments of time alone to simply think. You may not have a lot of extra space in your home, but with a little creativity, you can still create your very own mom cave, a customized retreat center designed especially for you. Ideally, it's nice to designate a whole room to be your mom cave, but few of us have the luxury of that much extra space. If you can't manage a whole room, try for a closet. If that's not possible, opt for a small table and chair, or a coffee table with a comfortable pillow or rug. You might consider an outdoor mom cave, designating an area of the patio, porch, or yard as your own special place.

Fill your mom cave only with things you enjoy. If your special place is outside, stow items in an airtight, waterproof container. You might include favorite books, some video games, a notepad and pen, instant coffees and teas, healthy treats, an MP3 player loaded with your favorite songs, or other things you enjoy. A blanket always makes a nice edition, as hiding beneath it creates an insta-cave and immediately surrounds us with a sense of comfort, warmth, and security.

Let others in your household know that when you're in your mom cave, you shouldn't be disturbed unless it's necessary. If you don't have that luxury, get up a little earlier or stay awake a little later so you can have some time just for you in your special place. Even five minutes of alone time can do a lot to relieve the stress and exhaustion that so often accompany motherhood.

Clutter: The Unwanted House Guest

It's one thing to keep your house clean before you have children and another thing entirely to keep it clean after you have children. A certain amount of mess just comes with the territory, and unless you're willing to spend every free waking moment of your day cleaning up or you're able to hire a professional cleaning service, chances are you're going to have to learn to live with a fair amount of clutter. The trick is to accept it and plan for it. By being prepared for clutter, you'll have easy ways to stow it out of sight and keep it reasonably under control so it doesn't take over your house or your life. When you have kids, clutter usually falls into one or more of the primary categories described here. Follow these tips to help keep clutter at bay as much as can be expected by any sane and reasonable parent who isn't the reincarnation of June Cleaver:

Toy Clutter

As your children grow and develop, they'll inevitably amass a large quantity of toys, some good, some not so good. Often, the toy supply is so vast that it becomes impossible to locate favorites and even see what all is available. With shelves and bins overflowing, it's tempting to do a major toy ditch, but at the same time, why get rid of a perfectly good toy that could potentially keep your child entertained for a while more?

Children's tastes and abilities change so quickly that it's not always clear which toys should be kept and which should be given away. Enter the rotating toy bin. Get a large plastic bin with a lid, possibly several if you have the storage space. Every month or so, fill the bins with items from your child's room that haven't been played with in a while. For older children, allow them to pick the items. Stow these bins in a closet or storage shed. When it comes time to rotate out the toys, return the items in the bins back to your child's room and fill the bins with fresh items. This is also a good opportunity to promote generosity while further reducing clutter by inviting your children to look through the bins to see if there are any toys they are ready to donate to a thrift store or charity.

In addition to the rotating toy bin, keep another bin or a basket with a lid in any other main area of your house where play generally occurs, be it the living room, kitchen, or play room. If you have unexpected guests or need to clean up in a flash, you can quickly throw scattered toys into the nearby toy bin.

Clothing Clutter

Another main clutter source for families is clothing. Clothes are constantly being outgrown, wearing out, and going out of fashion. Still other clothes are brand-new but are waiting to be grown into. Add to that the fact that kids can't seem to get anything out of a drawer without unfolding everything else in the drawer and it can seem like you're drowning in clothes. To keep the clothing river under control, sort through clothes regularly. If you're handy, keep a basket in the laundry area in which to stash stained or torn items for later repair, and choose a day each month to go through the basket. What can't be fixed can be reused for stuffed-animal making or other arts and crafts. If you're not likely to actually bust out a needle and thread or your stain removal arsenal, save yourself the bother and simply toss these dilapidated items in a clothing recycling bin, available in most communities. In addition, if you have clothes that don't quite fit yet or are out of season, store them out of sight until the time arrives when they can be worn. To keep children's drawers neater, roll up items rather than folding, and hang as much in closets as possible. Finally, don't keep anything you don't like to wear. If it doesn't make you feel good to wear it and it's not an absolutely essential item (like your only winter coat, for instance), ditch it. Donate it to a thrift store and maybe someone else will enjoy it.

Paper Clutter

Paper clutter is another major source of housekeeping woes. If you have school-age children, you'll find yourself continually bombarded with school papers, prized doodles, penmanship practice, and more. The best defense is to be ready. Keep some trays or baskets near your door so that school papers and other household paperwork can be sorted easily right when you get home. When dealing with school papers, you'll need to categorize them. Is it an informational paper about something that's going on at the school, an important date or time to remember? If so, transfer the relevant information onto a family calendar and toss the paper if you no longer need it. Is it a form you need to fill out, sign, or otherwise deal with? If so, put it in an action box or special folder designated for such papers. Is it homework your child needs to complete? Keep it in the backpack until they're ready to do it, then immediately return it to the backpack. You'll save a lot of time not having to look all over the house for the scattered remnants of your child's homework. Designate an art box for special drawings and other work your child has done that you would like to save for a keepsake. Once a month or so, transfer the drawings from the art box into scrapbooks or picture frames so you can enjoy them more easily. You might even arrange your child's art beneath the glass of a glass-topped coffee table for a creative display.

Think Twice Clutter-Banishing Charm

While this method certainly isn't foolproof, casting anti-clutter charms around your home's most mess-prone areas can indeed help keep the chaos under control. Face the space you want to protect, be it a living room end table or a kitchen countertop. Hold your hand with your fingers spread and extended and your palm facing the target area. Move your hand rapidly back and forth at the wrist, envisioning a white, silver, or lemon-yellow light emanating from your palm as you do so. Think of it as a pure, clear, clean light, and imagine this light flowing from your heart, through your hand, and into the target area. Imagine your family members approaching the area, ready to deposit keys, backpacks, papers, or other random items as usual, but see with your mind's eye the force field you have just created repelling these objects. Envision your loved ones thinking twice, stepping away from the clutter hotspot, and putting the items where they belong. If you like, seal the charm with the following words or a verse of your own creation:

Whatever touches cannot stay!
All items here are put away!
As I will it, as I say,
You will stay clean all day today!

A few times throughout the day when you're near the area, utter the following verse three times in succession to keep the charm strong:

Think twice, think nice.
The clutter is kept at bay!

Your Home, Your Way

In this chapter, you've explored lots of ideas for brightening your home and making it a place of magick. Let these ideas inspire you to add your own special touches to your home's décor. Whether it's an altar dedicated to Hecate or a shelf full of pig statues, the things you love deserve a special place in your home, just as you do. Take the time to make your home your own and it will become a space that supports you, sustains you, protects you, and recharges you.

Chapter 15

~~~~

Psychic Mama

Mothers need all the tools in their arsenals that they can hold, and one often overlooked yet invaluable asset is psychic ability. As a human, you have an inherent ability to perceive the astral and spiritual realms and to communicate with these energies on both a conscious and a subconscious level. You can practice this skill and train yourself to use this gift to great benefit. In this chapter, you'll learn some easy ways to enhance your natural sense of "mother's intuition," explore several tools to aid you in divining the future, and discover a ritual to help fully awaken your psychic abilities.

Mother's Intuition

Something happens at the moment you give birth. A new Spidey sense is ignited in your entire being and you have this profound sense of awareness that you cannot imagine until you experience it. You might find yourself waking up minutes before your baby wakes, your body's rhythms in perfect sync with your baby's. You might feel a sudden sense of uneasiness, followed moments later by the cries of your child who has just fallen and bonked their head. Mothers often feel a deep, inexplicable telepathic connection with their children, and for those mothers who are especially sensitive to psychic phenomena, this bond is even stronger and more apparent.

Mother's intuition is very real. Characterized by gut feelings and emotional, often instinctive reactions that seemingly arise out of nowhere, intuition actually has a scientific basis. Throughout our lives, we gather information about the world and the people around us. When we use our intuition, we're often basing our feelings on a culmination of past observations and experiences without realizing where the knowledge and information is coming from. This intuition can help you to solve problems, avoid danger, make ethical choices, and pick up on your child's feelings. Some intuitive experiences, however, defy logical explanation. Dr. Victor Shamas of the University of Arizona conducted a study of one hundred pregnant women all in their first trimester, asking them to intuitively predict the gender of their babies. A strong majority of 70 percent of the women were successful, crediting their accurate predictions to a mixture of gut feelings and prophetic dreams.[21]

It seems we mommies are hard-wired with a special connection to our babies, so trust in your mother's intuition and nurture it to the fullest. There are lots of ways to strengthen and improve your intuitive powers. Try the following tips and exercises to practice and hone your intuitive faculties. You may want to keep a log of your experiences so you can track your progress and identify your psychic strengths and aptitudes.

- Trust your instincts. If you have a wrenching, pressing feeling deep down in your gut, a persistent sensation that something is the matter or that someone is in danger, listen to it. Check on your loved ones to make sure they're okay, and be willing to change plans and adjust schedules if you feel it prudent to do so. While you don't want psychic phenomena to rule your life, you should not ignore your intuition. Uncomfortable, fearful psychic sensations usually turn out to be no real cause for alarm, but it's always better to be safe than sorry, so check it out before you dismiss it.

- Use it or lose it. The more you utilize your psychic sense, the more keen and reliable it will become. Everyone is born with a measure

21. Morgan Brasfield, "Mother's Intuition: Why We Should Follow Our 'Gut Feelings,'" Today.com, April 18, 2013, www.today.com/parents/mothers-intuition-why-we-should-follow-our-gut-feelings-1C9504706.

of psychic ability, but if you habitually ignore and seldom employ your intuition, your psychic sense will eventually wither and atrophy as a result.

- Keep a piece of them with you. By carrying around a lock of your baby's hair or one of their smaller garments such as a baby cap or sock, you'll have a physical object at hand that can serve to strengthen the psychic link between you and your child. When you can't be close by, handle the garment or hair while thinking of your little one. More often than not, you'll get an impression of what they're doing and how they're feeling, either through visions or through a feeling that seems to come from the heart rather than the mind.

- Carry intuition-enhancing herbs or stones, such as rosemary, sage, moonstone, or amethyst. When you feel that your psychic powers need a boost, hold the herb or stone in your hand and notice the flow of energy within it. Absorb this power into your core, then stretch out with your intuition and see if you get any further impressions.

- Anticipate and intuit. Observe your baby closely and try to anticipate your child's needs as much as possible. When your baby cries, use your intuition to quickly guess what the trouble is—i.e., a dirty diaper, hunger, tiredness—then test your instinct. A few seconds is all you need to tap into your feelings and make an initial assessment. If your instinct turns out to be wrong, try something else without delay. You'll likely be wrong plenty often, but the times when your first guess is correct will pay off in the way of fewer tears for you and baby alike, and your intuition will get stronger and sharper from the practice.

- Look into your child's eyes and hold their hands. What thoughts or emotions come to you? Think of your love for your child, and send this energy through your hands and into your child's tiny hands.

- If you have school-age children, place your hands on their backpack or jacket when they come home. What images come to mind? Do you feel a lot of positive energy or negative energy? Do you see your child engaged in any particular activities? What sort of day do you think your child had? Mentally make your predictions, then ask your child how their day went and what they did that day. In this way, you can show your kid you're interested in them, stay up to date about their feelings and experiences, and test the accuracy of your intuition, all at the same time.

- Practice your psychic skills with a pair of dice. Predict what number you will roll, then try to roll it. Track your successes and failures.

- To do a similar exercise with a deck of cards, place them all face down and attempt to psychically decipher which cards are hearts, which are spades, which are clubs, and which are diamonds. Divide the cards into four piles, one for each suit, then look at the cards and see how many you got right.

- Psychic power stems from our connections to the world around us, so get out in it. Spend plenty of time in nature, smelling the flowers, feeling the air on your skin, and touching the trees, the ground, and the grass. What do you sense?

- For an easy exercise to help awaken your psychic instincts and sharpen your mother's intuition, ask someone to place a piece of clothing from each member of your family on the table or floor, arranging them in a haphazard manner. Use clothing that has been worn rather than the freshly laundered stuff; you want your family's vibes to still be lingering in the fabric. Close your eyes and hold your hand an inch or two above the clothes. Can you feel any vibrations? Try to tune in. Can you identify who any of the clothing belongs to just by feeling the energy? Make your best guesses, then open your eyes and see how you fared.

- Whenever something is bothering you or you feel like you need information that can't be obtained through traditional means, give your intuition a shot at it. Think about whatever is on your mind and stretch out with your feelings. Don't direct your thoughts; allow them instead to flow naturally where they will. Are you surprised by anything you feel or envision? What does your heart tell you? Is your body filled with a pleasant, warm feeling, or do you feel anxious, with stomach tight, jaws clenched, and skin crawling? When you turn off or at least turn down your conscious thought process, your physical body and subconscious mind will speak to you loud and clear.

Divination Tools for Mothers

When intuition isn't cutting it, try a little old-fashioned divination. Divination, more crudely and commonly known as fortunetelling, is useful for a variety of purposes, from gaining insight into problems to discovering the location of lost items. Practicing divination is also a great way to hone your psychic abilities and sharpen your natural intuition. Here are a few divination methods to try, along with some ideas for how a mother might employ each one. If any appeal to you, investigate further and start experimenting and exploring until you feel comfortable and familiar with the particular tool you're using. While predictions are never set in stone and accuracy is rather variable, once you've got the hang of it, divination becomes increasingly reliable, insightful, and effective.

Pendulum

A pendulum is a divination tool consisting of a string or chain with a heavy bead, crystal, or other small weighted object attached to one end. The string or chain of the pendulum is held firmly between the thumb, forefinger, and middle finger so that the weighted end of the pendulum hangs straight down. Simple yes or no questions are then directed at the pendulum. With your arms and hands held completely still, you wait for the pendulum to begin its motions, and from there, you decipher the answers.

While pendulums can't provide detailed information, they certainly can help you assess the possibilities of various circumstances or situations. For instance, you might ask your pendulum, "Is my baby a girl?" or "Will this new job suit me well?" The pendulum will begin to swing either back and forth or in a circle to reveal its answer. Traditionally, a back-and-forth motion is said to indicate a negative response, a circular motion is taken as a positive response, and an ambiguous or mixed motion indicates that the matter can't be answered at present, but your own workings with the pendulum might prove quite different.

Before you pose a question to the pendulum, test its swings so that you will be able to determine what each type of motion means for you personally. To do this, simply hold the pendulum suspended over the open, flat palm of your other hand, and ask the pendulum to show you in turn what "yes," "no," and "uncertain" look like. You may also want to pose to the pendulum a question to which you definitely know the answer, to check the pendulum's accuracy. For instance, if you're wearing a red shirt, you might ask the pendulum, "Is my shirt blue?" Then see if it answers correctly. A pendulum is not 100 percent accurate by any means, but it can definitely provide reassurance and guidance when you've got something on your mind.

You might also use a pendulum to help locate lost or hidden items, which is a very helpful technique for a mom to know. If you're new to motherhood, you won't believe the number of socks, shoes, homework papers, backpacks, and hairbrushes that will vanish at the worst possible time, usually about five minutes before you need to rush out the door. In such times, take your pendulum into each of the likeliest areas where the missing item might be located. Ask the pendulum, "Is it in here?" Then await the response. When the pendulum gives you a positive response, start searching. You can let the pendulum guide you more directly by simply letting it hang down and noticing from which direction you feel a pull.

It's important to note that pendulums are easily influenced by the subconscious mind. If you're not feeling objective, don't use a pendulum, as it will only tell you what you want or expect to hear. You might find it helpful to cast a circle around your space and clear your head before you begin your pendulum divination, as this will ensure you're surrounded with good energy and in a mind frame conducive to psychic work. Simply envision the space you're in encompassed by a glowing, positively charged, pure light. Imagine all the negative energies in the area clearing out of the space. Try to sense these energies and direct them out and away from the area. If you like, petition additional help and guidance from any deities or other spiritual entities with which you like to work.

If you don't have a pre-made pendulum, you can easily make your own. Take a nine- to twelve-inch length of fishing line, hemp twine, or any other kind of string and tie something fairly heavy to the bottom. You might use a bead, a crystal, or a metal washer. If you're using a very thin and delicate string such as thread, you can even use a sewing needle to act as the pendulum. If you like, attach a smaller, lighter-weight bead or crystal a couple of inches or so below the top of the string. Leave enough room to tie a loop at the very top of the string a half inch or so above the optional smaller bead or crystal so the pendulum is easier to hold. Be sure your pendulum hangs straight down and is evenly balanced.

Tarot Cards

A deck of seventy-eight cards used for divination, the tarot employs eso-teric symbolism and universal archetypes to reveal and interpret infor-mation originating from the psychic or spiritual realms. Tarot cards can provide greater detail and more specifics than can a pendulum, as each card in the set conveys its own complete story through imagery. There are many books available offering advice and information on how to read the tarot, but don't discount your own natural intuition and in-stincts. If you're able to tell a story from a picture, you're able to read the tarot. Let each image speak to you, and listen. What do you notice first about each card? What feelings does it give you? What images and thoughts occur to you as you gaze at this card? The same card can mean different things to different people in different readings, so each card represents a range of possibilities rather than one single definite truth. It's up to the person doing the reading to decipher through intuition and knowledge of the tarot what message each card is conveying in any given situation.

You may wish to bless and energize your tarot deck before you use it. One way to do this is to wrap it well in a piece of natural fabric and bury it in the ground under the light of a full moon. Leave the deck in the earth for two days and then retrieve it. If you like, anoint the deck with a small drop of your blood or saliva before you bury it to ensure that it's fully in tune with your own unique essence.

Whenever you need insight or specific guidance, try pulling a card or two out of your tarot deck. What does the image say to you? Consult at least two different tarot guides to cross-reference card meanings, and decide for yourself what the likeliest interpretation is for each card. You might also do a simple three-card reading, pulling one card to represent what has been, one card to signify what is now, and a final card to represent what is to come.

The tarot can be a very helpful tool in deciphering the hidden emotions and motivations of children, especially once they reach the secretive teenage stage. Direct communication with your child is, of course, the best option for finding out how they are doing, but if you just can't shake the feeling that something is amiss even though they're saying everything is fine, check it out with the tarot. Think about your child and the specific matter at hand, ask your question, and pull as many cards as you feel called to pull. You might ask things like "What is my child really feeling now?" or "Is my child telling the truth?" or "What can I do to help my child?" Keep your questions specific and action-oriented, and don't get too upset by any negative imagery that might come up in the cards. The tarot speaks in extremes and ambiguities, so look at it from a tempered perspective. Ultimately, keep in mind that the tarot has its limits. To get a full and more accurate picture of any situation or circumstance, there's simply no substitute for direct communication.

Oracle Cards

Often much simpler and much more positive overall than tarot cards, oracle cards follow no set standard or structure. Oracle decks can be found in a multitude of themes and designs, from cat-themed oracles to fairy-themed ones. Many people find oracle decks easier to read than the tarot, as the cards are usually less complex and more straightforward. Typically, a new oracle deck includes an instruction book detailing how to use the deck and offering suggestions for how each specific card should be interpreted.

If you're looking for some extra encouragement to help you through the daily demands of motherhood, or you're worried and you need some reassurance, an oracle deck is an excellent choice. Ask the cards, "What can I look forward to today?" or "What can I focus on to make this a great day?" or "What resources do I have to overcome this challenge?" Oracle cards tend to offer an optimistic outlook, so they're an ideal choice during pregnancy and while your children are very young, when you don't really need all the complexity and potential darkness that the tarot can reveal. If you're prone to paranoia and suspicion or you're not too confident in your psychic skills, a positively themed oracle deck would likely be a better choice for you than the tarot.

Ritual for Awakening and Enhancing Your Psychic Abilities

To fully awaken your psychic sense, try this ritual. On the night of the full moon, go outside with a bowl of water and a piece of moonstone. Hold the bowl so that you can see the moon's reflection in the water. Think about the energies associated with the moon, its intuitive, subtle nature, and its ability to illuminate the darkness and shed light on what's hiding in the shadows. Envision these energies flowing into the water.

Next, hold the moonstone up toward the sky so the moonlight can shine directly on it, filling it with lunar power. Dip the moonstone in the bowl of water, right in the middle of the reflected moon, then touch the stone to your forehead in the area of the third eye chakra, located between your eyes and about an inch up from the top of the bridge of your nose. Feel the lunar energies flowing into you, then recite the following verse or say something in your own words to express your intentions:

Moonlight, moon bright, lovely moon I see tonight,
Make me just as wise and bright!
Bless me with your hidden light!
Let me share your awesome sight!
My psychic mind is strong and bright!

Keep the moonstone close whenever you're performing psychic work, or simply tuck it in your pocket every day if you want to sharpen your intuition 24/7.

Chapter 16

Beautiful Mama

We're all familiar with the stereotypes, demands, and expectations placed upon the 1950s housewife. Not only were women expected to keep the house spotless, handle childcare, and prepare hot meals for everyone in the household, but they were also expected to pull off the miraculous feat of looking fabulous while they did it.

Fortunately, modern women have largely escaped these outdated and unrealistic expectations, yet somehow we still feel a little guilty at times for not being able to meet these ridiculous standards. We want it all—the successful career, the successful home life, the successful personal life—and as modern women, we can have all that. It's not necessary, expected, or required that we look our best every day while simultaneously playing the roles of working mom, super mom, and super woman, but when we do manage to look great while we're managing everything else, it helps us to feel empowered, beautiful, confident, and in charge. Beauty and style are not something to do for others. They are concepts you can embrace for yourself that will allow you to shine every day like the star you naturally are, and feel good every minute of it.

We mothers face a whole lot of "ugly" every day, from dirty diapers to dirty laundry to dirty dishes. It may seem pointless and even stupid to strive to look good while dealing with an endless number of nasty chores, but if you make an effort to do so, you will find the unpleasantries of motherhood much less unpleasant. By putting even a little time into caring for your appearance, you will begin to remember what it feels like to feel beautiful, and you will reclaim a lot of your personal power in doing so.

Motherhood is great, but let's face it: we get lost in it. What mother has honestly not spent a day without even once dragging a brush through her hair or bothering to change out of those worn-out pajamas? What mother's underwear drawer can honestly compare to her pre-motherhood one? Sexy lingerie gets replaced with more practical and comfortable plain cotton undies, and money that was once spent on expensive bra and panty sets is now spent on diapers and onesies.

We begin to put our children first in everything we do, and we start associating personal luxuries and self-pampering with selfishness. There's no good reason for this. There's no bible that says mothers have to wear ugly, worn-out, geriatric-style underwear, right? No manual that proclaims all good mothers should look as frazzled as they feel, right? While we should and we do make our children our number-one priority, there's absolutely no benefit to your children in you going around looking all frumpy and frazzled, and absolutely no harm will come to them if you take a little time to make yourself feel good and look more beautiful. Reclaiming your pre-motherhood sense of beauty and style can be a challenge, though, when you have so very little time to spare, so in this chapter, we've put together a few ideas to help you get started.

Beautify Your Aura

When you feel beautiful, you look beautiful, and when you *don't* feel beautiful, you can fake it till you make it with a little magick. Glamour doesn't come from the clothes you put on but rather flows out from your aura, which can be altered and tailored to suit your mood just as easily as you might take up the hem on a favorite skirt to match the times. In fact, the word *glamour* is derived from an early Scottish term used to describe magick spells and enchantment; it implies an illusion, a certain haze or charm that can be cast about oneself. When you're consciously projecting an aura of beauty, people around you will see you as more beautiful, and soon you'll begin to see yourself as more beautiful, too.

To create your own glamorous aura, simply stand in front of the mirror and look at yourself, just as you are. Pick out one feature that you like and focus on its beauty. Adjust your posture and see how it affects your appearance; stand up straight, lower your shoulders, tilt your chin slightly up, and smile. Think of how loving and kind your soul is, and let this energy flow out from your heart to surround you—envision it as a glowing bubble of warm, rose-colored light. Say to yourself, "I am beautiful and I radiate an irresistible aura of glamour and appeal!" As you go about your day, continue to hold yourself and move about as if you were one of the most beautiful creatures on earth, and when you catch yourself slumping, correct your posture and repeat the affirmation.

Dress for Luck

Each of the twelve signs of the zodiac has its own lucky colors. Incorporate your own lucky colors into your wardrobe choices to help increase your sense of inner harmony and attract more good luck into your life. Follow the guide here to get you started. These colors need not dominate your outfit; a simple accessory or two in the chosen color will be enough to attract good vibrations.

For Aries: Black and red are your luckiest colors for fashion. Try maroons, burgundies, and dark charcoal grays for variation. Splashes of green and yellow might also be used.

For Taurus: Pale pink, yellow green, deep blue, and indigo are your lucky fashion colors. Experiment with shades of rose, olive green, and forest green, too.

For Gemini: Yellow, light green, shimmering silver, and white fabrics resonate well with you. Try a dash of orange here and there as well.

For Cancer: White, silver, and emerald green are the best fashion choices for you. Experiment with shades of ivory, cream, jade, and jewel green, too.

For Leo: If you want to dress for luck, yellow, orange, gold, and white are the best options. Try your sunniest yellows and metallic golds to enhance your solar qualities to the fullest.

For Virgo: Green, blue, yellow, gold, white, or light gray clothing works well for you. Incorporate various shades of these colors into your outfits to help bring out your natural power.

For Libra: Blue, purple, green, and yellow are your luckiest fashion colors. Try balanced shades that are neither too light nor too dark to best align with your levelheaded personality.

For Scorpio: Dark reds and browns make you shine. Experiment with maroon, crimson, mahogany, and shades of rich chocolate brown as well.

For Sagittarius: The best fashion colors for you are orange, purple, and blue. Try wearing clothing in shades of bright blue, bright or burnt orange, indigo, and plum to bring extra luck into your day.

For Capricorn: Gray, purple, brown, and black vibe well with you. Also try shades of beige to rich, deep brown; lightest grays to darkest grays; and vibrant purple, indigo, or lavender.

For Aquarius: Blue and green are your luckiest shades. Try vibrant, bright, even electric hues to enhance your natural magnetism.

For Pisces: Purple and sea green are your luckiest clothing hues. Try lavender, violet, plum, and various shades of pale green as well.

When You Can't Get to the Spa, Go to the Fridge

It's a lucky mother indeed who has the luxury of post-baby trips to the spa or salon. For most of us, it's hard enough to get five minutes to ourselves, much less an afternoon, not to mention the fact that the cost of expensive beauty treatments can be prohibitive when faced with the rising price of diapers, clothes for the children, food for the family, and other necessities more pressing than a pedicure. When you need a little pampering but you don't have the time or the money to spend on an all-out spa service, don't let yourself feel neglected. Just try some do-it-yourself methods to enjoy salon treatment at home.

You don't need a lot of expensive ingredients, nor do you need a ton of time. Just head to your refrigerator, raid your cupboards, and then lock yourself in the bathroom. A good ten to twenty minutes is all you need to emerge feeling beautiful, pampered, and refreshed. Try these homemade spa treatments and see how simple beautiful can be:

Oatmeal and Sugar Scrub

Feeling a little rough around the edges, like, literally? Try scrubbing yourself down with this all-natural exfoliant to remove dull, dry cells on the surface of your skin. Just mix equal parts white sugar and raw oatmeal, moisten it with a small amount of warm water, and rub the mixture over your arms, elbows, knees, and legs. Remove the excess with a wet washcloth, then hop in a hot shower to finish hosing down.

Spa-Style Facial

Why not treat yourself to a complete facial just like you would get at a real spa? Begin by steaming your face to open the pores. Just heat some water on the stove and hold your face a comfortable distance from the steam, allowing the moist, hot air to penetrate your skin. Next, use your favorite face mask. Slather on a thin layer and allow it to dry. After you rinse off the mask, exfoliate. This will help smooth away dull skin cells and remove any residuals left behind by the mask. Follow with a gentle cleanser, then use a toner such as witch hazel. Simply moisten a cotton ball or washcloth with the toner and rub it over your face and neck. Finally, moisturize using a good facial cream. Night creams work well, as they are often thick in consistency and highly concentrated. For affordable and all-natural facial products, check out the beauty aisle of your local natural food store or try out your own do-it-yourself recipes.

Avocado and Banana Moisturizing Mask

Dry, tired skin tends to sag and wrinkle, making you look older and frazzled. Revitalize your skin with a super moisturizing mask made from ripe avocado and fresh banana. Place half an avocado and half a banana in a sturdy bowl, then mash them with a fork until evenly blended and smooth. Test the blend on a small section of skin on the inside of your arm and wait thirty minutes to an hour to be sure you don't have any allergic reactions or sensitivities. Spread the mixture on your face and let it sit for about five to ten minutes. Wipe off the excess with a washcloth, then rinse your skin with warm water followed by a final splash of cold water to help close your pores and seal in the moisture.

Honey and Olive Oil Hair Fix

If your hair tends to be dry and frizzy, try this monthly conditioning treatment to add moisture and seal in shine. Mix ½ cup warm honey and two tablespoons olive oil, then rub the mixture into your hair, paying special attention to the ends of the hair shafts. Leave on for about ten minutes, then rinse hair thoroughly.

Cider and Beer Hair Shine

To make your hair softer, silkier, and shinier, mix equal parts beer and apple cider. Let the mixture sit until it's room temperature, then pour on washed, wet hair. Leave on for about five minutes, then rinse carefully and follow with your favorite conditioner to remove any lingering odor from the cider and alcohol.

Beautifying Baths and Showers

Being clean and well groomed is the most essential aspect of looking your best. Even when you're busy, make time for regular baths and/or showers, and make the most of them. When you take a bath, use it as an opportunity to scan your body and assess your emotions. Are you stressed? Do you need to shift your focus? How does your physical body feel? Is anything hurting? Focus on the sensations you're experiencing, and if there is anything unpleasant, envision these energies seeping out of your body and into the water to be neutralized and balanced. As you get out of the bath, imagine your body as pure, filled with a radiant light and beauty that shines brightly for all to see.

Another easy way to help yourself become more beautiful inside and out when you take a bath is to use a special combination of stones and crystals to enchant the water with a balancing, harmonious energy that will help you feel and look your best. Place onto a small square of fabric a piece of bloodstone, a clear quartz, an amethyst, a rose quartz, and a fluorite. Tie the rocks securely in the fabric to make a little bundle that can be placed directly in the bathwater. As you take your bath, think about the energy of the stones enhancing your beauty and supporting your overall health and well-being.

For the shower, you might consider creating a body scrub made of fine-grain sea salt or Epsom salt mixed with jojoba, grapeseed, or hemp oil and a drop or two of lavender essential oil. Sea salt is known to help pull toxins and negative energies out of the body, while Epsom salt helps soothe sore muscles and relax the physical body. If you like, use a balanced blend of both salts. Put a dab of the scrub on your washcloth or loofah and rub gently over the surface of your skin in smooth, circular motions. As you do so, you can rid yourself of a lot more than just dead skin cells; let any negative thought patterns drift into the water to be washed away as well. Use your time in the shower to explore and enjoy your body. Connect to yourself. Appreciate yourself.

Self-Acceptance Is the Key to Beauty

While beauty tricks and miracle products abound, the most important and effective thing you can do to look your best is to cultivate self-confidence and self-acceptance. If you're feeling bad about yourself, you will actually be less physically attractive. And there is no reason you should ever feel bad about yourself. Each and every one of us has our own beautiful traits, our own brand of shine that makes us sparkle. We also all have qualities that we're likely to perceive as faults.

Do your best to let go of any negative feelings about yourself and your body. Pregnancy can certainly do a number on us, as can life in general, but bodies come in all shapes and sizes and all are beautiful in their own unique and wonderful way. Find the beauty in yourself and focus on it. Realize that no one else will notice your so-called flaws as much as you do, if they even notice them at all, so don't let any minor imperfections get in the way of allowing yourself to feel great.

Chapter 17

~·~

Sexy Mama

Sex after motherhood (or while pregnant) is a whole different ballgame than sex *before* motherhood. No longer are there countless hours of leisure in which to plan and prepare for romance; no longer does putting on sexy undies feel so reasonable. After a day spent immersed in baby duty and mommy tasks, your fantasies are more likely to be in the realm of reading a book in your pajamas than in making hot, primal, passionate love. We need this, though. As a woman, you need it. And your partner, if you have one, needs it too. It's a challenge to do so, but if you don't make the effort to keep your passions alive, you'll find yourself faded, frustrated, and jaded before you know it. Mommy or not, you're a sexual creature, and you deserve to honor that side of you. Here are a few tips to keep the romance and passion in your life alive and kicking.

Long Live the Quickie, Even if It's Rather Short

So you might not have hours to spend in foreplay, and you don't have the luxury of being as loud or wild as you once were before tiny listening ears filled the house. But you can still have fun with yourself or with your partner, even if you have only a few minutes. Though the days as a parent are filled with activity from start to finish, there are those precious moments scattered throughout—five minutes of peace and quiet sprinkled in here or there while the baby is napping or is being watched

223

by another caregiver. Take advantage of this free time, however short it is. Sneak away somewhere private and touch yourself or your partner. You don't have to get *too* hot and heavy, as you'll probably have to go right back to mommy duty, but just allow yourself to enjoy the moment and experience some moderate titillation. On the other hand, if you feel you have adequate time and you do want to take it further, just lock the door, turn on some music, and have at it. Sure, sex is better when you have all the time in the world, but it's still great even if you have only a few minutes. A quickie with yourself or with your partner will work wonders in keeping your sensual side thriving.

Sacred Sex

Now, when you *do* have the luxury of more time to spend with an intimate partner, there's a lot you can do to really make the most of it and enjoy connecting not just physically but spiritually as well. The main difference between "just sex" and sacred (or spiritual) sex is the connection made between the body and the spirit. One way to start activating and utilizing this connection is to explore your partner as fully as possible with each of your senses, as often as you can.

Taste

Taste your partner. Rub your tongue not just in their mouth or even in the sexual areas. Truly *taste* your partner. Use your tongue to explore your partner's body. Lick your partner's lips and feel each crack and fold of their mouth. Use your teeth to feel the texture of their skin in certain areas. Light nibbling is very sexy around the nipples, the earlobes, the tops of the shoulders, and even the knees. Don't use the touch of your hands or your vision as part of this exercise. Use only your mouth. Taste your partner fully.

Touch

In each of your fingertips lie some of the densest nerve endings on the body. Through the hands and fingers you can send messages to your partner without saying a word. One exercise that can help you connect very deeply with your partner is to sit face to face and place your hand over your partner's heart while they place their hand over your heart. Put your other hand over their hand that is now over your heart, as they do the same with their other hand. Allow the energy of your heart to pulsate into your partner's palm, and feel the energy they send to you.

Another way to focus on touch is to explore your partner's body using just a fingertip. You might touch your partner's lips, chest, genitals, or any other mutually agreeable place. Wherever you touch, you're setting into motion a multitude of physical and energetic reactions in your partner's body as well as your own. Now touch your partner with your whole hands, exploring their body all over as you convey to them your love, letting your deepest thoughts and feelings for them flow from your fingertips and into their skin. Receive the energy from your partner's reciprocal touches, and allow yourself to get lost in sensation.

Smell

As you and your partner draw closer and your bodies begin to move and come together, you begin to release pheromones, the chemicals and smells of sex. *Your* sex. The smell that is created and smelled only by you and your union with this particular partner. How intimate is that? There are lots of ways to utilize your sense of smell during a steamy bedroom session. In addition to appreciating the naturally occurring "sex smells," try using aromatic candles or scented oils to add fragrance to the room and create a more sensual vibe. Select a scent that makes you feel relaxed or aroused. Here are some essential oils that are believed to enhance arousal and sensuality.

Anise: Anise smells a lot like black licorice and is believed to arouse lust, especially in women.

Jasmine: Jasmine has a light, floral scent that most people find very appealing. It has been used in India for many years to improve sex drive and inspire arousal.

Neroli: Produced from the bitter orange, neroli is a sweet, citrus scent with slightly metallic undertones that is believed to help increase the female libido.

Sandalwood: This heady, earthy scent works great for inspiring a man's passions, but it should never be applied directly to the skin, as it can cause irritation.

Vanilla: Vanilla is said to increase a man's attraction to a woman and is considered by many to be a powerful aphrodisiac.

Ylang-Ylang: Ylang-ylang helps alleviate sexual frustration by enhancing arousal, relieving stress, increasing pleasure, and improving the overall mood. It has a strong, exotic floral scent. Too much exposure can cause headaches, but when used in moderation, the scent of ylang-ylang is sensual and lovely.

A great way to use these oils is with an aromatic oil warmer. It comes with a small space for a tealight candle, and there is an open bowl on top for water and drops of the essential oil to burn while the candle is lit. It's sexy and smells delicious and is not too strong since the oil is diluted. Many oils can also be used directly on the skin, but some oils, such as sandalwood and cinnamon, can cause skin irritation if they're not heavily diluted. Always use natural (not synthetic) essential oils that are recommended for use on the body, and test each oil in small quantities to make sure you don't have any sensitivity to it. If irritation develops, wash off the oil and discontinue use.

Sound

Through sound, a romantic ambiance can be established in an instant. Music is a great way to set the tone for lovemaking. You might choose a song that you associate with sex or romance, or simply choose something relaxing to help you let go and get in the mood. You can also use sound to set your intentions with your partner. Use your words to express your feelings and desires to your partner, and listen closely as your partner does the same. Tell your partner you love them, tell them the things you want to do to them. Maintain eye contact with your partner and speak kindly, deeply, and honestly so they'll feel comfortable sharing their own intimate wishes and emotions.

Sound also plays a major role in the actual physical intercourse part of sex. While no one wants to carry out an entire conversation while making love, it's beneficial to let your partner know through words or other sounds what feels good to you. Through our most intimate sex noises, we communicate with our partners in a way that becomes a private language. If you do a specific moan when you reach a certain level of pleasure, you don't have to explain yourself. Your partner hears that sound and knows that they are onto something good, that they are in the area of choice. They are doing what feels good to you, and this boosts their confidence, which in turn boosts your own pleasure. A confident lover is a better lover, so use sound to your advantage to let your partner know when they are doing something just right.

You can also utilize sound to help you and your partner synchronize your breathing patterns. Put your foreheads together and breathe deeply into each other. Take in your partner's breath, receive it, and return it. Let the energy of each breath circulate throughout your bodies. The breath creates a higher union between you and your partner; use this and ride the energy of it into your lovemaking experience. As you bring your lips together to kiss, breathe fully into each other. Keep your breathing at a similar pace. The breath will guide your entire experience, all the way up to the moment of orgasm where the toes curl and for a moment the breath ceases and then explodes with might and energy. The breath is your guiding force throughout. It becomes hot, loud, and heavy as passions rise. Use the magick of sound to embrace your sexual experience and help you enjoy it to the fullest.

Sight

Sight can be a great asset to your sexual experiences. Look into each other's eyes and use your sight to connect completely. Observe your partner's body throughout the process and try to see beyond their skin. Use your sense of sight to help you determine what your partner is feeling and experiencing. Don't overanalyze anything. Simply observe. See yourself and your partner in this sacred space, and appreciate all that you observe around you. Use your eyes to enter into your partner and experience them in a new and deeper way.

The Sixth Sense and Sex Magick

In addition to touch, hearing, sight, smell, and taste, many people acknowledge a sixth sense. This is the sense of intuition, or psychic ability, which allows us to experience and interact with the universe in ways that transcend and transform physical reality. Utilizing the sixth sense during sex helps take the experience far beyond the physical level and into the realm of spirit, where real magick can happen. Sex is not only fun, but also fuel—fuel for our passions, fuel that can make our wildest dreams come true. If you want your sex to be truly sacred, use it as a springboard to take you and your partner to heightened states of awareness. Utilize it to help you connect to each other and to something much bigger.

Sex is truly magickal, and you can use it to accomplish great things. Try this little exercise in sex magick and see for yourself. You'll be using your sixth sense throughout this process, so approach this with an open mind and trust your instincts. Get your partner on board as well, and select a common goal or intention that you would like to pursue together, be it a new home, greater prosperity, greater intimacy, a healthy child, or whatever else you wish for. As excitement builds between you and your partner, allow yourselves to visualize a common goal: see in your minds the two of you enjoying absolute success. When climax is achieved, imagine all the energy built up between you and your partner bursting into the wider universe, ready to help rearrange reality in a way that brings you closer to the success you desire.

If You're Not Getting What You Need, Give It to Yourself

While all this sacred sex stuff is lovely, let's be honest and upfront here. Whether we're without a partner, or whether we have a partner and they're just not doing it for us as much as we'd like, there are times when we must take our sexual pleasure into our own hands, literally. Sex is a human need and lust a very enjoyable human condition. Even busy moms can and should enjoy them both. If you don't feed your passions, these aspects of yourself can quickly fade away, leaving you feeling dumpy, frumpy, and all "mommed out," for lack of a better phrasing. We start to feel like mommy machines, existing only to protect and serve, only to please others, and we are expected to see our own pleasure as our absolute lowest priority.

Don't fall into this trap. A mother can still be a whole person, a whole woman with all her sensual aspects and powerful passions fully in place and energized. When you're honoring your whole self, you feel happier, more whole, more loved and loving...and that is something every single one of us totally and completely deserves. Allow yourself some fantasy and sensuality in your life. Do what you can to express your passions, whether it's through art, writing, making music, or simply daydreaming. See yourself as the sexy woman you want to be, and become that. You don't need anyone else's approval or participation to enjoy some sensual excitement. Pamper yourself, love yourself, touch yourself. Insist on making time for yourself, and use that time to unwind and open your heart and mind to greater love, passion, and excitement.

The Great Escape

Try this next time you're bummed out about having to do a chore like washing the dishes or anytime you can steal a few minutes alone (the bath is a great refuge). Continue doing whatever other activity you happen to be doing, but allow your mind to wander to a fantastic scene. Envision yourself someplace very romantic, very sensual. You see a person beckoning to you, someone you find completely and impossibly attractive. This could be a real person you personally know, a made-up person of your own erotic creation, or even a celebrity you secretly crush on.

Let the scene develop in your mind. Enjoy the details of sound, sight, and touch. If you're alone, go ahead and touch yourself a little. Stroke your arms and neck lightly with your fingertips. Let your fantasies carry you as far as you like, or as far as your limited time allows. When you've finished with your fantasizing, place your hand over your heart and say out loud or to yourself, "I am beautiful and sexy, and I deserve this in my life!" What you're doing with this action is transferring your emotionally charged thoughts into intentions, which in turn transforms your passionate energies into real-life opportunities for passionate pleasures.

Fantasy is a powerful tool. By imagining something, it opens the door for the imagined something to actually manifest. Enjoy your fantasies and passionate desires, and think of them as magick in the making.

Look Sexy, Feel Sexy

It's nearly impossible to feel sensual when you're wearing last year's ratty underwear and oversized pajama pants. Even though it might feel silly, allow yourself the luxury of dressing to feel and look your best. Of course you won't want to put on your finest attire to clean up baby puke and mop the kitchen, but you can still make an effort to keep your appearance relatively neat and up to date. You don't have to have a lot of money to be fashionable. Thrift stores, consignment shops, and yard sales can yield fabulous fashion finds, as can setting up a clothing swap night with friends or neighbors. Get rid of anything you own that's stained or torn, or if you're crafty, trim off the bad parts and transform your old clothing into something new.

Personalizing your fashions with colors and accents that reflect who you are and how you're feeling can be a lot of fun, too. Try bright colors when you're feeling happy, playful, or outgoing; pastels or muted tones when you're feeling serene or romantic; darker shades when you're feeling introspective, thoughtful, or rebellious; and whites when you're feeling radiant.

Remember also that even though you won't want to wear revealing clothing around your children, you can always wear some super-sexy lingerie beneath your everyday attire. You might even give your partner a peek at what you're wearing underneath. Having this little secret can spice up your day by stirring your passions.

Top Ten Stones for Love and Romance

If you want to invite more love and romance into your life, try making use of the powerful earth energies found in naturally formed stones and crystals. Each stone has its own unique vibrational pattern, and the energy of certain stones can be harnessed to attract greater love, romance, intimacy, passion, and harmony. Here are ten such stones that lovers around the world and throughout the ages have found beneficial in increasing intimacy, promoting harmony, and opening the heart for love. Heart-shaped stones and soulmate stones—fused stones composed of two or more stones joined together—are also lucky.

Amethyst: This stone promotes passion and attracts love.

Aquamarine: Associated with long-lasting love, this stone is believed to protect the bond between lovers and is especially beneficial when partners must be apart.

Blue Lace Agate: This stone has a calming, peaceful vibe that promotes harmonious communication and encourages loving feelings.

Emerald: This stone is beneficial in strengthening partnerships and promoting fidelity.

Green Aventurine: This stone brings luck in love and helps create more opportunities for romance.

Jade: This stone is believed to attract love and inspire romance. It's also a symbol of lasting love and loyalty.

Lepidolite: This stone encourages peaceful interactions and harmonious relationships by lessening stress and protecting against outside negativity.

Moonstone: This stone increases feelings of love and passion, encourages honesty, and promotes unity.

Rose Quartz: This pink variety of quartz crystal is especially beneficial for promoting love and attracting romance.

Turquoise: This stone is great for increasing intimacy, encouraging friendship, and promoting feelings of harmony between lovers.

Using Stones for Love and Romance

Carry any of the stones in the previous list with you, wear as jewelry, or place near the bed to attract new opportunities for love and romance. You might consider procuring a set of matching stones, one for you and one for your partner. To empower your passion-boosting stones, simply hold them in your hands while thinking of the love you wish to give and receive. Let this energy flow into the stones. If you like, place them under the light of a full moon to help strengthen the charm.

Chapter 18

Kid Magick

As a magickal mom, you probably want your kids to be magickal, too. From psychic games to magickal crafts, there are lots of ways to encourage your growing child to value and develop their own intuitive and spiritual potentials. In this chapter, you'll find some ideas for incorporating psychic development into playtime, discover several magickal crafts to make together, and learn how to cast a simple charm to help soothe away the distress of those all-too-common minor boo-boos that children are so prone to get.

Kids are naturally in tune and in touch with the spiritual world, and they are born as psychically intuitive, sensitive beings. All we have to do as parents is to not get in the way of that, and to offer opportunities for these skills to be utilized and developed. You won't be able to use most of the ideas in this chapter until your kids are well out of the baby stage, but if you expose them to the world of spirit and start nurturing their natural abilities as soon as possible, they're not as likely to lose those connections. Read on to see how you can continue to incorporate magickal experiences into your child's life as they continue to grow.

Hide and Don't Seek

Show the child a certain toy or object and then go hide it. Then ask the child to close their eyes and imagine in their own mind where you put it.

Encourage them to use their psychic ability and intuition to find the object. Don't let them just jump up and go searching right away. Help them visualize and imagine and intuit where the hidden object might be. Once they have a hunch of where to look, let them get up and search. If they are way off, you might guide them into the correct room or provide other hints until they are able to pinpoint the object—or get bored and give up. Keep it fun, lighthearted, and playful as you encourage your child to develop their abilities. Let them believe in their psychic powers, and it won't be long till those abilities flourish in earnest.

Pick-a-Crystal

Take about five or so crystals and show the child all of them. Choose crystals of different varieties, such as smoky quartz, rose quartz, citrine, clear quartz, and amethyst. Make sure the crystals are large enough that the child can't choke on any of them if they are still at a stage where they put things in their mouth. Encourage your child to touch and play with the crystals. Let them get to know the energy of each crystal, and then take the crystals away for a moment. Have the child close their eyes, then place one crystal in the palm of their open, flat hand. Tell them to keep their eyes closed, but see if they can tune in to the energy of that crystal and tell you which one it is.

As a variation, pick one of the crystals and let your child "charge" it, holding it in their hands and filling it with loving, happy vibrations. Just tell them to hold the stone and think of something happy or something they love, and then send their energy into the crystal. Next, mix the crystals back together, have your child close their eyes, and place the crystals on their palm one by one, asking them with each crystal if that's the one they charged.

Psychic Coloring Game

Get some crayons and a coloring book and ask your child to select a page for you to color. Let your child look at the image for a moment, then ask them to close their eyes while you color something in. With eyes still closed, ask them if they can guess which color of crayon you used and what element of the picture you colored. For instance, did you color the doggy yellow? Or did you shade in the lady's hat blue with pink polka dots? Take turns and see how many correct picks you can make. You might start with just a few color choices, then incorporate more crayons as you get in more practice and sharpen your psychic skills.

Touch the Trees

Touching trees is another wonderful way to encourage your kids to explore the magick and energy of the world around them. Let them feel the various energies of different trees. Let them sit at the bottom of a tree and look up, let them hug the trees, let them feel the bark and the leaves. Let them try to stand like trees. Go to a park or wild area and show your children different trees like maples, oaks, or pines. Have them place a hand on the tree and ask them to notice what the tree feels like, what kind of energy it seems to have. After trying this with a few different trees, ask them to close their eyes. Lead them by the hand to touch one of the trees, or perhaps a different tree of one of the same species. Ask your child if they can tell you which type of tree it is, just by feeling its energies.

Go Barefoot

Going barefoot, also called "earthing," is a great method for staying in tune and in touch with the grounding, nurturing, strengthening energies of Mother Earth. If you're somewhere safe where the ground is free of pokey objects, encourage your kids to go barefoot. Ask them if they can feel the energy of the earth climbing up through the soles of their feet to help nurture their spirit and ground their bodies.

Magickal Rattle Crafting

Rattles have gone hand in hand with both magick and babies for thousands of years. As varied as they are versatile, rattles come in countless shapes and sizes. Used for raising good energy, chasing off negative energy, or simply making some noise, this percussion instrument makes an easy-to-use and fun first magickal tool for kids.

It's easy to make your own magickal rattles, as long as you keep the design fairly simple. Rattles tend to contain small objects that pose a choking hazard for children under three, so your best bet with kiddos this age is to buy a ready-made rattle designed especially for babies, then charge it up with your own loving intentions and magickal power. Older kids over three who are well past the choking hazard stage might make their own special rattle. One simple method is to begin by giving your child a paper cup and asking them to decorate it with markers or stickers. They might write their name, draw a picture of themselves, draw pictures of things they love or that make them happy, or draw pictures of things they think of as powerful, which could be anything from Santa Claus to the sun to a dinosaur. Let your child be creative.

Next, have your child choose some beans, rice, seeds, beads, or other small objects to put inside. Place whatever rattle contents they've chosen in a bowl, and ask them to stand beside it or hold it in their hands. Invite your child to think about the kind of things they want to do with their rattle. Ask them to imagine having fun with it and to let the energies of these thoughts drift down into the bowl. Let your child pour the objects into the cup, then help them cover the top with a circle of construction paper. Tape securely around the cup's circumference to keep the rattle's contents from escaping. If you like, let your child place the rattle under the sunlight or moonlight for an hour or so to charge it and get it ready for magick.

Another slightly more complex rattle design that older kids might enjoy is the sistrum. Ask your child to find a stick that's shaped like the letter Y—something smooth, not sharp, and with a fork at one end. The stick should be anywhere from six to ten inches long. Once they've chosen the stick, have your child hold it up toward the sky to invite the powerful energies of sun and air to enter into it. Next, invite your child to select several beads, metal nuts or washers, soda pop tabs, old keys, or any other small object that will rattle and has a hole in it. Have your child hold their hands on the objects they've selected and think about the energies they want these things to impart to the rattle. Ask them why they chose these objects and have them describe what each object reminds them of. For instance, there might be a yellow bead that reminds your kid of the happy sunshine, or a soda pop tab that reminds them of the excitement and pleasure of special treats or special occasions. Don't press your child too much; let them put things in their own words, and if you like, ask questions to gently encourage them to elaborate.

Next, attach a piece of wire or heavy twine to the Y shape at the end of the stick. Tie one end of the wire or twine securely onto one of the two prongs. Have your child string their chosen beads or other objects onto the twine or wire, imagining as they do so what it will feel like to shake the rattle and play with it. Then tie the other end of the wire or twine securely to the second prong. When the rattle is done, invite your child to shake it, dance around with it, and laugh out loud to get it energized and ready for action.

One nice use for a magickal rattle is to use it to chase away worry, fear, bad dreams, gloominess, and other unpleasant feelings. It's important to encourage your child to acknowledge and express their feelings, and it's also good to give them some tools for getting out of a slump when they're ready. Let your child know that whenever they're feeling sad or fearful or worried, they can, of course, talk to you about it, and they can also shake their magickal rattle to help chase away the negative energy. Have them shake the rattle very hard and vigorously to start while they shout out loud for the negative energy to go away. They might shout out, "Go away, bad dream!" or "Go away, sad!" Let them put their problem into their own words and express in their own way how they want that problem solved. Tell your child to slow and soften the pace of the rattle once they feel the bad energies clearing out of the area.

Magickal Paper Planes and Helicopters

Another fun craft to do with kids is to create your own set of magickal paper planes or helicopters. Simply create your paper aircraft in whatever fashion you choose, from the most basic to the most complex design. You can find how-to instructions online for a variety of simple-to-make designs. Once you've constructed your plane or helicopter, it's time to make it magickal. Ask your kid if they have any special wishes, and ask them to draw pictures, words, or symbols on the wings of the aircraft to represent these wishes. For instance, a row of happy faces might be used to symbolize more friends, a picture of a teddy bear might represent a wish for more toys, or a simple star shape might be used to symbolize any wish. Ask your child to think of their wish as they decorate their flying vehicle. Once the airplane or helicopter is complete, have your child express their wish as you launch the paper aircraft toward them in a symbolic act of bringing them exactly what they desire. You may want to make your own magickal aircraft, too, and invite your child to try to land it on you as you lie flat on the floor and smile up at that precious giggling face.

DIY Fairy Garden

If your child is interested in fairies or other nature spirits, invite them to make their very own fairy garden. They sell pre-made fairy garden kits at many toy stores, but making your own is more fun, more affordable, and far more magickal. Simply choose an area of your yard or a large flowerpot to be the location of the fairy garden. Fill the pot with good soil, or if you're doing this right in the yard, loosen the dirt to get it ready for planting. If you're making a yard garden, you might consider placing a perimeter of stones or sticks around it to help delineate the area. If you like, add a little bit of glitter to the dirt to give it that sparkly touch that fairies are known to love. Next, have your child poke some little holes in the soil using a gardening tool or their fingers. Let your kid choose some seeds to plant. Dried beans, marigold seeds, or grass seeds tend to have an excellent success rate and grow quickly. Have your child put the seeds down into the holes and then cover them with soil.

Next, add more special touches to your garden to help attract the fairies. Invite your child to add anything they can find that they think the fairies might like, such as shiny rocks, decorative stones, sparkly costume jewels, seashells, large or colorful leaves, or pretty flowers. Your fairies are bound to get hungry and thirsty, so choose a couple of lids taken from milk jugs or soda bottles to act as the food dishes. Fill one with water and the other with dandelions, honey, sugar, strawberries and cream, or other treats your child thinks a fairy might like. For a special touch, have your child choose some pieces of tree bark, twigs, stones, or other natural objects to act as furniture for the fairies. An empty nut shell might make a nice little chair, while a hollowed-out orange half filled with water or leaves might make a nice bathtub or bed.

Once the fairy garden is constructed, have your child water the seeds daily. When the plants begin to grow, you'll know that fairies must be afoot. Visit the garden in the evenings or early mornings, and ask your child if they notice anything unusual. Does it look like the plants are growing right before your eyes? Does it look like any of the fairy furniture has been moved or rearranged? Does it feel as if tiny invisible wings may have just rushed past your head? Is there a trail of flower petals or tiny footprints in the dirt? Try blowing some bubbles near the garden. Do they seem to drift in odd directions, as if something very tiny could be hitching a ride on the bubble stream? These things may be evidence of fairy activity. If your child isn't noticing any fairy action, invite them to ring a bell by the garden to help call the fairies near, then have them sit quietly in the shadowy evening light and see if they sense anything. Fairies seldom come right out in the open; they speak to us instead in whispers, signs, symbols, subtle movements, and feelings.

Bubble Wishes

Blowing bubbles is fun for people of all ages, and it can be a versatile and wonderful vehicle for magick, too. Try having your kid charge the container of bubbles with all the happy energy they can muster. Then have them make a wish with each blow. As the bubbles drift up in the air, they'll carry the wishes with them. You might even make colored bubbles, aligning each wish to a corresponding color. For instance, you might use pink bubbles for love, or blue or yellow bubbles for happiness. To color your bubbles, just add a small amount of washable paint to the bubble solution and shake well. This is best done outdoors, for obvious reasons. You might blow the bubbles onto pieces of paper or canvas to create your own bubble art.

Tear Jar

We all need to cry every now and then, whatever our age. It can be very healing to let those tears out. At the same time, we don't want to cry forever, and we certainly don't like to see our children crying for very long. If your child is upset and you've talked about it but they're still having trouble stemming the flow of tears, try distracting them from their gloom with a tear jar. Any clean jar with a lid will do. You might even make a label that says "Tear Jar." Put in the jar a piece of turquoise and/or a piece of citrine to add peaceful, comforting energies to your creation.

When your child is crying, tell them to hold on a minute, that you have to go get something. Bring in the tear jar and tell them you don't want all those tears to go to waste. Hold the jar gently against their cheek under their eye and ask them to cry you up some more tears to fill the jar. If they ask you what you want them for, just say something vague and mysterious, like tears are good for watering the weeping willow tree, for example. Your child will likely stop crying very quickly once the tear jar comes out. Just look inside it, shake your head, and say something like, "Well, I guess that's good enough for now, if that's all the tears you have. Let's go have some fun." Put the jar away out of sight and get back to enjoying the day.

Boo-Boo Soothing Charm

While serious injuries always warrant prompt and professional medical attention, your child is bound to get a variety of lesser scrapes, bumps, and bruises that require nothing more than perhaps a bandage and some good old-fashioned motherly love. When your child has a very minor injury but is acting like it's the most horrible pain ever, try this simple boo-boo soothing charm.

Hold your hand above the injury. Don't touch it, but instead just hover over it. Try to tune in to your child's energies. Move your hand back and forth and notice the difference in how the energy from the injured part feels in relation to the feeling you get from the surrounding skin. Can you feel heat or a sort of sharpness or tingling? This is the pain or infection. Move your hand as if you are drawing this energy out and away from your child's body. Pull those painful energies up into your palm, hold them tightly in your fist, then shake your hand vigorously while you say or think "neutralize!" Touch your hand flat on the ground to deposit the lingering energy, or shake your hand over a bag or box to later be thrown away. Repeat this until you feel you have drawn out as much of the painful energy as possible.

Next, you want to infuse the injured area with soothing, healing energy. Shake your hands to get them fresh for this next stage, then spread out your fingers and think about a lavender-tinted light made of pure healing energy coming into your hand. If you like, ask any spirits or deities you believe in to help bring you this healing energy. Once you can feel that energy sitting right there in your hand, hold your hand over your child's injury again, and with your palm open and your fingers slightly cupped, direct this energy into your child's body, moving your hand slowly back and forth above their skin as you deposit the healing light. Wash your hands after this so that all that energy of pain and discomfort you just dispelled won't cling to you. Your child will be feeling better in no time.

Chapter 19

Powerful Mama

A mother is a special being, a giver of life, love, wisdom, protection, and all the millions of other things for which our children come to rely on us. Filling such a tall order is a lot of work, and the constant demands and high expectations of motherhood can be exhausting and overwhelming. It's very easy to lose our sense of self, to feel like our sole purpose in life is to serve others, to be "just a mom" and nothing else.

To talk about being "just a mom" is a ridiculous notion, of course, as a mother is often the whole world to so many. Yet you are much more than a mother; you are also a woman, a magickal person, and an individual with your own hopes, dreams, talents, and interests. Each and every one of us has a spectacular light, a certain spark of creativity, passion, and compassion that not only fuels our own soul but also has the power to light up the world.

When we do our best to nurture our gifts, feed our passions, and honor our own truth, that light within us shines so clearly and brightly that the universe will often conspire to manifest our greatest schemes and grandest dreams. This chapter will show you how to do just that. Through a series of exercises, rituals, and visualizations, you will discover your own inner power and learn how to connect to that power and activate it to achieve your full potential both as a mother and as a unique human being otherwise known as *you*.

The Empowered Mother

As a mother, you will have so many jobs. It might be incredibly difficult to find time for yourself beyond being a mother, and if you have another career on top of that, it's so much to handle. For a time, you might completely lose yourself—and it's perfectly natural and normal to lose yourself in the experience when you welcome a new precious baby into your life. What's not okay, however, is to *stay* lost in it. You can't become a mom and try to be a wife and maintain a career and leave nothing left over for your own hopes and dreams. If you make that mistake, you'll find yourself feeling increasingly drained, depressed, and unmotivated.

We mothers tend to feel selfish if we continue to pursue our own desires, and that's just silly. We teach our children by example, so if you don't make the time to show your kids that you matter, they can end up picking up this same limiting belief about themselves. Honor your own inner light and your own brightest dreams. Before you were a mom, you were *you*, and even as your priorities shift to the demands of parenthood, you can still be the you that you are meant to be. This goes beyond getting out of the house to do something nice for yourself. This is serious. This is about finding your soul's purpose and honoring that purpose—not only your purpose in being a mother, a wife, or whatever else you might be, but also your soul's truest calling, the passion inside you that you want to express and share with the world. If you've always had a dream, even if it seems farfetched, don't give up on it just because you've become a mom. You can't ever ignore that fire inside you, and in fact you must fuel it to the fullest.

You don't have to have huge dreams. They don't need to bring you fame or fortune. They just need to ignite your passion and keep you the incredible, sexy, strong, divine person that you are. If your passion is photography, get those pictures, mama. If it's writing, always make time to write anytime the creative flow enters. If it's to teach something, go! Do it. Put yourself out there. If your passion is to do art or music of any kind, by all means, get to it and make it yours.

Try your best to let your children be part of your dreams and your passions, but make time to do these things on your own as well. If you want to go within and do something wonderful all by yourself, honor that creative flow and go for it. Children learn so much more by what we show them than by what we tell them. Whatever dreams and aspirations you have for your children, make sure to share some of that energy and desire with yourself, too. If your kids see that you honor your own talents and pursue your own best dreams, they'll know it's not just words you're speaking when you urge them to do the same. Everyone has the right to pursue their own personal goals and passions, so give everyone in your home permission to feel alive, creative, joyful, strong, passionate, determined, and able. Show them by your own example that this is a home where inspiration is followed and dreams come true.

If you haven't yet figured out what your true calling is, try this simple meditation to help you awaken to your soul's grander purpose:

Soul's Purpose Meditation

Close your eyes and imagine yourself as the most empowered, wonderful, successful, spiritual, and sexy version of yourself. Sit with this thought; let the images swirl and evolve in your mind's eye. Does this vision of your ideal self come easily to you, or does it take a while for the images to formulate? Visualize this best version of yourself in as much vivid detail as possible. What do you look like here? What type of activities are you dressed for? Where are you, and what do you see? What are you doing? Are there other people near you? What other things do you notice? Stay with this image for as long as you like, and try to remember everything you see.

When you open your eyes, write down exactly what that image was. Then evaluate what you saw or sensed in the meditation. Who were you there, and what exactly were you doing there? Contemplate your vision and try to figure out what sort of dreams or passions you might have that would make sense with that scene. Were there photographers around you in the scene? Perhaps you're meant to try a career in modeling, acting, music, or something else that might make a person famous. Were you surrounded by delicious fresh foods in an expansive and pristine kitchen? Perhaps your path will lead you to the culinary arts.

Decipher your vision to the best of your abilities, and repeat this exercise once a week or so until you've developed a very clear image of your very best self. The next step is to ask yourself this big question: Are you doing anything in your daily life to help make this image of your ideal self a reality? If so, what are you willing to do next to follow this dream all the way through? If you're not currently pursuing this goal, ask yourself why not. Challenge any limiting beliefs or doubts you might have by giving yourself a shot at it. You'll never succeed if you don't try, so identify one solid step you can take every day or every week to start making your dreams a reality, and just do it.

Helping Is Key

Deciding who or what you want to help or how you want to improve the world is a huge key in discovering your dreams, making it happen, and unlocking your full potential. Do you want to help monkeys in the rainforest? Or would you perhaps like to help victims of domestic violence to find healing? Maybe you want to bring fresh drinking water to impoverished or drought-ridden areas, or perhaps you would like to improve the health of our oceans and help protect them for future generations. Figure out who or what in life you most want to help, or what you most want to accomplish. Determine the impact you want to make with your existence—the best, most awesome ways you might imagine sharing your love, energy, ideas, effort, and talent with the world.

Once you get that part down, all you have to do next is brainstorm ways in which you might use the talents, skills, and abilities you already have to help you accomplish your bigger, overall goal. For instance, do you want to help save animals and you happen to have artistic talent? If so, why not make some art to sell and donate a portion to an animal sanctuary, or use the money to help pay your way through veterinary school? Do you have good speaking skills and a passion for bringing happiness to children? Consider becoming a professional storyteller.

That simple first step of figuring out who or what you want to help will illuminate the many paths forward to achieve your greatest dreams and grandest potentials. There's another happy bonus, too. If you have a goal to help someone or something other than yourself, you won't be as likely to feel selfish in pursuing your goal to the fullest and dedicating time to it. When others are invested in our success, we have more built-in motivation because it's not just ourselves who will miss out if we don't do whatever it is we have in mind. If you want to do something good in the world, that becomes more important than insecurity, more important than doubt, more important than fear. Get clear about your goals and know exactly why and for what purpose you want to accomplish them. By aligning yourself and committing yourself to your greatest visions of success, you'll find that motivation, inspiration, and opportunity come naturally.

The Sacred Flow of the Universe

If you're pursuing your dream of being an artist, a writer, or anything else that lends itself to creativity, the universe will conspire to let you in to this new way of being. You might call it "entering the flow." When you enter the flow, things line up and you begin to change from deep within. You become aligned to your highest will, and that highest will in turn becomes aligned with the sacred flow of the universe. Your creativity will flow more readily, and opportunities will pop up where you least expect them when you are using your talents in ways that harmonize not only with your very best, truest self, but also with the world itself.

As you begin to transform from the inside out and go after your dreams with gusto, you will encounter two kinds of people: the ones who believe that you are capable of going so much higher than you ever thought possible, and the ones who are not comfortable with you changing and expanding. Those people in the latter camp will naysay everything and appeal to the part of you that wonders, "Why me? Why do I think I could do something so special? Who do I think I am, anyway?" Other people will appeal to the inspired part of you that thinks, "Why *not* me? Why shouldn't I live an extraordinary life? Why shouldn't I have everything and more than I've ever wanted?" Surround yourself with encouraging, loving, inspiring people. Let go of the naysayers and go with the flow.

Reach for the Stars Ritual

Here's a simple ritual that will help you attract the resources into your life that you need to succeed. Go outside, preferably under a starry sky and barefoot. Stand with your feet planted firmly on the ground. Stretch one arm up at a time, alternating arms as you reach toward the sky. Spread your hands and fingers out wide. Imagine something that would help you feel more empowered in your life. It might be courage, prosperity, knowledge, or another resource. Reach up and act as if you are grabbing on to this resource; close your fist around it and hold on to it. You might visualize it as a shining star that is now in the palm of your hand. Bring this hand down and place it over your heart, opening your palm and slowly rubbing this good energy right into your heart chakra. Now reach up with the other hand and repeat the same process, reaching up for different things each time. It might be something as simple as a comforting thought, an affirmation, or a simple stroke of good luck that you're after. Whatever it is, reach up and grab it tight.

When you've finished reaching for the stars, rub your hands down the length of your body, starting at the heart and moving down to the torso, pelvis, legs, feet, and right down to the ground beneath your toes, mixing heaven and earth with your own sacred intentions.

Ritual for Success

For this success-bringing ritual, you'll need a piece of paper and something to write with, a cup of water, a candle, and a stick of incense. Do this ritual after you've decided on a major goal you'd like to accomplish. This could be your life's mission, or a lesser goal, but pick something big that you truly care about and truly want to achieve. Write this goal on the piece of paper, along with the reasons and motivations that make you want to accomplish this feat. State it all in assertive, positive terms. For instance, if your goal is to become a nurse to help heal people and relieve suffering, you might write something like "I will be a nurse and I will heal people and relieve their suffering" as opposed to phrasing it as "I hope to one day become a nurse because there are many hurt and sick, suffering people." State that you *will* do whatever it is, rather than stating that you *want* to do it. The phrasing does indeed make a big difference in this particular act of magick.

Once you've written down your goal, take the paper outside and lay it flat on the ground. Place your hands flat on the ground at each side of the paper so that your hands are touching both the bare earth and the paper. Envision these powerful earth energies flowing into your goal, charging and fortifying your intention. Next, sprinkle some of the water onto the paper. Envision cleansing, quenching rains showering down on your goal, giving it new life and nourishment. Light the candle and place this above the paper. Visualize the warm sun heating your goal and magnifying the power of your intention. Finally, light the incense stick in the candle flame. Move the incense over the paper, making a pentacle shape as you visualize the power of the air element moving your goal forward swiftly and certainly. Plant the incense stick in the ground below the paper so that the candle flanks it at the top and the incense flanks it at the bottom. Just keep them far enough away so none of the hot wax or incense ashes will fall onto the paper.

Read your goal out loud and feel in your heart what it will be like to have accomplished this. Feel that success; imagine it and bring it clearly into your heart and mind. Finish by uttering the following verse, or simply say a little prayer or affirmation in your own words:

> *Powers of earth! Bring strength to my goal!*
> *Powers of water! Bring life to my goal!*
> *Powers of fire! Ignite my goal!*
> *Powers of air! Move swiftly my goal!*
> *Earth, water, fire, air!*
> *You will help me, if I dare!*
> *True to my goal, I will stay!*
> *Please bring me what I wish today!*

Keep the paper tucked in your pocket or purse, or place it on your altar. If part of your goal is to enjoy greater prosperity, anoint the paper with bayberry oil and carry it in your wallet.

The Rainbow Technique

This exercise connects the energies of the solar plexus to the heart on the inside. The solar plexus is the region that receives emotion and drives confidence, will, and ambition, while the heart is the steady provider of a loving, pulsating power. Aligning these two regions of your body will help you heal any emotional hurts that you may have experienced, and also help you realize what a special, wonderful, mystical being you truly are.

Place one hand on your heart and the other hand over the solar plexus chakra, located above the navel. Take some deep, calming breaths. Try to use your breath and your intention to connect the energy like a rainbow from one hand to the other. Imagine the rainbow as a loving, nurturing energy. Try to first feel the rainbow on the inside of the body, arcing inward through your body from hand to hand. Once you feel this connection, you can form the rainbow of energy into a full circle that now goes outside the body, too. Feel the rainbow of energy pass through your hands. Do this for as long as it takes to feel connected and warm from one hand to the other, and breathe comfortably and rhythmically in sync with the sacred vibe now circulating through you. If you practice this exercise regularly, you'll find it easier to feel loved, to be loved, and to be love. You'll discover confidence and charisma you never knew you had.

The Lion

If you want to be a lion, you've got to learn to play like one. This exercise will assist you in releasing any pent-up tension to help you get back to being your truest, most powerful self. Sure, it looks very silly, but who cares? Let your kiddos or other family members have a good laugh and let them get in on the action if they want. Start by clenching your jaw (not too hard, though) and pursing your lips. Close your eyes and tighten the muscles in your face to intensify this. Then open your mouth as wide as you can, stick your tongue out as far as you can, and let out a loud sigh on the exhale. As you exhale, don't just sigh; release. Release any stress, tension, or fears that you are experiencing but don't want to admit to out loud. You don't have to put these fears and anxieties into words. Just simply breathe them out with every exhale.

Do this several times, then take a few deep, steadying breaths. When you're ready, think about all the great qualities you have, then let out a tremendous roar! Embrace your lion-heart instincts and become fierce.

Top Ten Stones for Success and Personal Empowerment

Here are the top ten stones to use to help you attract success, achieve your goals, and feel confident and awesome while doing so.

Aventurine: Attracts prosperity, brings career success, and opens new avenues.

Carnelian: Boosts motivation and increases courage.

Citrine: Citrine is one of those "good for just about everything" stones. It promotes success, improves confidence, and increases good luck.

Garnet: Improves confidence and encourages ambition.

Jade: Improves leadership ability, enhances authority, and attracts wealth, success, and opportunity.

Lodestone: Attracts resources and opportunities.

Moonstone: Brings new beginnings and good fortune and aids in creative pursuits.

Orange Calcite: Helps remove creative blocks and boosts confidence.

Ruby: Increases courage, improves leadership ability, enhances authority, brings inspiration, and attracts prosperity.

Tiger's Eye: Brings personal empowerment, courage, and vision.

Using Your Stones for Success

There are many ways to use stones to attract success. You might choose one or several of the stones in the previous list and simply carry them with you in a pocket or purse, incorporate them into a special piece of jewelry to wear daily, or keep them close whenever you are taking an important step toward achieving your goals. For instance, you might bring your stones with you to a job interview or tuck them into your pocket while you create your next artistic masterpiece.

You can also use your success stones to impart extra magickal power and luck by rubbing them directly over items related to your goal. For example, you might rub your success stones across the surface of a job application, or if your dream is to be a professional tarot reader, you might keep a sampling of success stones right in your tarot bag so that their energies will be imparted to the cards. You might keep your success stones on your altar, along with something to symbolize your specific goal, be it a stethoscope to represent dreams of practicing medicine or a pen to represent dreams of being a journalist. Handle your success stones often, especially when you feel your confidence or motivation slipping into a slump.

Healthy Self, Happy Self

Once you welcome children into your life, your eating habits are likely to change drastically if you're not careful. You might be so busy mothering that you forget to eat entirely, or you might find yourself eating leftovers off your child's plate more times than you'll want to admit. Sleeping patterns are also interrupted, and sleep is no longer several hours in succession. If you don't make a point of eating and sleeping properly, you'll have no energy left over for exercise, which is equally important and equally challenging to fit into your life as a mom.

Maintaining an exercise program or yoga practice when you have babies or small children in the house is an exercise in itself. It's not that you can't do it; it's just that it won't look the way it did when you had only yourself to tend to. With a young child or baby around, your exercise habits will inevitably change, bending into a new form. If you make an effort, though, and cultivate persistence and flexibility, you can totally pull it off, and you'll feel stronger, healthier, and happier as a result. Here are some tips to help you incorporate exercise, yoga, or other healthy practices into your busy life as a mom:

• Find the right practice for you. If you don't already have a practice that moves you, don't just go with whatever exercise regime is the latest trend. Do some research and find a practice that really moves your soul, whether it's martial arts or yoga or dance.

- If you're not able to take a regular class outside the house, simply practice on your own at home when you can find time. Video resources abound that give step-by-step instructions for a variety of healthy ways to get active.

- Don't be too attached to the idea of trying to have a set daily time for exercise. Exercise is likely to be squeezed in during one of two fairly unpredictable times: when your little one is sleeping or when they're happily playing and entertaining themselves. Try to take advantage of such times. You might put some toys near your exercise mat so you can do your thing with your child right there beside you. If you're not able to fit in your exercise practice during these times or you prefer a more regular schedule, you might try waking up earlier or staying up a little later and do it then.

- Expect interruptions. Don't be too attached to the idea of doing your whole exercise routine from start to finish. If there's a wee one around, chances are you'll have to press the pause button every now and then. When life hands you a stinky diaper, stop and change it— and then get right back into your fabulous groove.

- Accept distractions. In yoga, it's taught that what we might think of as "distracting"—like a loud TV or a child's noisy toy, for instance—is all part of the natural flow that you should invite and welcome in rather than try to tune out. Go with the flow, whatever that flow may currently be. Don't fight it, but instead invite the sounds, the distractions, and the perceived chaos into your practice and let it be an assistant in uncovering your own divine sense of inner peace. Look at it as a challenge to stay calm and focused on your exercise practice even if your toddler is taking the moment to press the siren button on his toy fire engine—again and again and again. With practice, patience, and determination, you can definitely do it.

Motherhood and the Art of Self-Care

Whether you are pregnant now, are trying to get pregnant, just had your baby, or already have several children, you must treat yourself right. If you are not in the habit of treating yourself well, you are missing a major component of general good living. You absolutely must give yourself the care and love you deserve. If this doesn't come easily to you, don't give up. Practice, and soon you will develop new habits that help nurture and honor your truest, best, healthiest, happiest self.

Self-care begins by finding ways to put yourself first. It doesn't have to be all day long, but it can't be never. Try to take at least a little time for yourself each day to pursue your dreams, interests, and passions and to sustain your physical well-being. You might even use this time to try some of the visualizations, exercises, or other ideas in this chapter. Remember that children learn what they see. If you have dreams and you put them off to the side to raise children, those children will miss out on learning about the magick of following your dreams. If you teach your children that you don't matter as much as everyone else, they will wind up doing the same. Just like your child, you are special. You are a one-of-a-kind, living, loving, conscious part of the universe. You are your child's guide, your child's protector, your child's mother. *You have to matter.*

References

Ainu Museum. "Child Rearing," in "Ainu History and Culture." www.ainu-museum.or.jp/en/study/eng11.html.

Alexander, Laurel. *Natural Wellness Strategies for Pregnancy*. Forres, Scotland: Findhorn Press, 2012.

Allured, Janet L. "Women's Healing Art: Domestic Medicine in the Turn-of-the-Century Ozarks." Bernard Becker Medical Library Digital Collection. http://beckerexhibits.wustl.edu/mowihsp/articles/Ozarks.htm.

Bird, Debbie. "Pregnancy Customs." BabyWorld. October 1, 2011. http://posts.mode.com/pregnancy-customs.

Brasfield, Morgan. "Mother's Intuition: Why We Should Follow Our 'Gut Feelings.'" Today.com. April 18, 2013. www.today.com/parents/mothers-intuition-why-we-should-follow-our-gut-feelings-1C9504706.

The Breastfeeding Center. Recipe based on "Housepoet's Famous Lactation Boosting Cookies." Massillon, OH, www.thebreastfeedingcenter.com/files/46628276.pdf.

Cielo, Astra. *Signs, Omens, and Superstitions*. 1918. Reprint, Pomeroy, WA: Health Research, 1969.

Costa, Shu Shu. *Lotus Seeds and Lucky Stars: Asian Myths and Traditions About Pregnancy and Birthing*. New York: Simon & Schuster, 1998.

Franklin, Rosalind. *Baby Lore: Superstitions and Old Wives Tales from the World Over Related to Pregnancy, Birth, and Baby Care*. Burgess Hill, UK: Diggory Press, 2005.

Frazer, Sir James George. *The Golden Bough*. New York: Macmillan, 1922; Chapter 21, Section 11, "Knots and Rings Tabooed," www.bartleby .com/196/54.html.

Gruber, Rebecca. "Baby Gifting Traditions from Around the World." Popsugar. July 23, 2013. www.popsugar.com/moms/Baby-Gift -Traditions-Around-World-31022688.

Haines, Cynthia Dennison, MD. "The Vivid Dreams of Pregnant Women." WebMD. www.webmd.com/baby/features/vivid-dreams -of-pregnant-women.

Lynch, C. D., R. Sundaram, J. M. Maisog, A. M. Sweeney, and G. M. Buck Louis. "Preconception Stress Increases the Risk of Infertility." *Oxford Journal of Human Reproduction* (March 23, 2014). doi:10.1093 /humrep/deu032.

Maity, Pradyot Kumar. *Human Fertility Cults and Rituals of Bengal: A Comparative Study*. New Delhi: Abhinav Publications, 1989.

Meyer, Melissa. *Thicker Than Water: The Origins of Blood as Symbol and Ritual*. New York: Routledge, 2005.

Monaghan, Patricia. *The New Book of Goddesses and Heroines*. St. Paul, MN: Llewellyn Publications, 1997.

Pattanaik, Devdutt. *The Goddess in India: The Five Faces of the Eternal Feminine*. Rochester, VT: Inner Traditions, 2000.

Poulsen, Anders. *Childbirth and Tradition in Northeast Thailand: Forty Years of Development and Cultural Change*. Copenhagen: Nordic Institute of Asian Studies, 2007.

Primal Trek. "Chinese Marriage Charms." http://primaltrek.com /marriage.html.

Rogan, Jim. "Armenian First Tooth," in "Local Legacies." The Library of Congress. http://lcweb2.loc.gov/diglib/legacies/loc.afc.afc -legacies.200002748/.

Tapp, Nicholas. "Hmong Religion." The Chinese University of Hong Kong. https://nirc.nanzan-u.ac.jp/nfile/1512.

Totelin, Laurence M. V. *Hippocratic Recipes: Oral and Written Transmission of Pharmacological Knowledge in Fifth- And Fourth-Century Greece*. Leiden: Brill, 2009.

Wedding Things. "Traditional Sri Lankan Buddhist Wedding Customs."
    http://weddingthings.lk/83-articles/latest-news/72-traditional-sri
    -lankan-buddhist-wedding-customs.

Williams, E. Leslie. *Spirit Tree: Origins of Cosmology in Shinto Ritual at
    Hakozaki*. Lanham, MD: University Press of America, 2007.

Index

To Write to the Authors

If you wish to contact the authors or would like more information about this book, please write to the authors in care of Llewellyn Worldwide Ltd. and we will forward your request. Both the authors and publisher appreciate hearing from you and learning of your enjoyment of this book and how it has helped you. Llewellyn Worldwide Ltd. cannot guarantee that every letter written to the authors can be answered, but all will be forwarded. Please write to:

Melanie Marquis and Emily A. Francis
℅ Llewellyn Worldwide
2143 Wooddale Drive)
Woodbury, MN 55125-2989

Please enclose a self-addressed stamped envelope for reply,
or $1.00 to cover costs. If outside the U.S.A., enclose
an international postal reply coupon.

Many of Llewellyn's authors have websites
with additional information and resources.
For more information, please visit our website at
http://www.llewellyn.com

GET MORE AT **LLEWELLYN.COM**

Visit us online to browse hundreds of our books and decks, plus sign up to receive our e-newsletters and exclusive online offers.

- **Free tarot readings • Spell-a-Day • Moon phases**
- **Recipes, spells, and tips • Blogs • Encyclopedia**
- **Author interviews, articles, and upcoming events**

GET SOCIAL WITH **LLEWELLYN**

Find us on 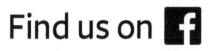 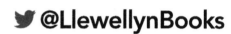 @LlewellynBooks

www.Facebook.com/LlewellynBooks

GET BOOKS AT **LLEWELLYN**

LLEWELLYN ORDERING INFORMATION

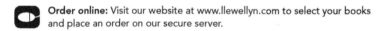

Order online: Visit our website at www.llewellyn.com to select your books and place an order on our secure server.

Order by phone:
- Call toll free within the US at 1-877-NEW-WRLD (1-877-639-9753)
- We accept VISA, MasterCard, American Express, and Discover.
- Canadian customers must use credit cards.

Order by mail:
Send the full price of your order (MN residents add 6.875% sales tax) in US funds plus postage and handling to: Llewellyn Worldwide, 2143 Wooddale Drive, Woodbury, MN 55125-2989

POSTAGE AND HANDLING

STANDARD (US):
(Please allow 12 business days)
$30.00 and under, add $6.00.
$30.01 and over, FREE SHIPPING.

INTERNATIONAL ORDERS,
INCLUDING CANADA:
$16.00 for one book, plus $3.00 for each additional book.

Visit us online for more shipping options.
Prices subject to change.

FREE CATALOG!

To order, call
1-877-
NEW-WRLD
ext. 8236
or visit our
website

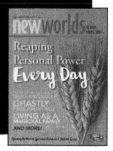

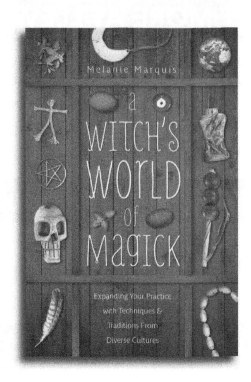

A Witch's World of Magick
Expanding Your Practice with Techniques & Traditions from Diverse Cultures
Melanie Marquis

This sparkling, in-depth examination of theories and techniques from around the world will help you reach higher levels of magickal insight and success. Each chapter features examples of tried-and-true magickal techniques gathered from the annals of folk magick around the world. By becoming more familiar with these classic "magickal moves," you'll have a solid starting point for designing your own mystical innovations.

Melanie Marquis, author of *The Witch's Bag of Tricks*, helps you explore the ins and outs of magickal skills and concepts from an eclectic perspective, providing a deeper understanding of spellwork and a greater appreciation for our magickal world. From Wiccan spells to Chaos magick, magick without tools to potion-making, discover love spells, word charms, curse-breaking, potion-making, contemporary spellwork, and more.

978-0-7387-3660-0, 240 pp., 6 x 9   **$16.99**

MELANIE MARQUIS

the
witch's
bag of
tricks

PERSONALIZE YOUR MAGICK & KICKSTART YOUR CRAFT

The Witch's Bag of Tricks
Personalize Your Magick & Kickstart Your Craft
Melanie Marquis

Increase your power, improve your spellcasting, and reclaim the spark of excitement you felt when you took those very first steps down your magickal path. The first book of its kind to offer solitary eclectics a solution to the problem of dull or ineffective magick, *The Witch's Bag of Tricks* will help practicing witches renew faith, improve abilities, and cast powerful spells that work. Whether your rituals have become rote or your spells just aren't working, you don't have to settle for magickal mediocrity!

Designed for the experienced eclectic practitioner, this guide offers advanced spellcasting techniques and practical hands-on exercises for personalized magickal development. You'll gain the skills and knowledge you need to custom design your own spells and advance your mystical development. Breathe fresh life into your practice and take your magickal skills further than ever with *The Witch's Bag of Tricks*!

978-0-7387-2633-5, 264 pp., 6 x 9 **$17.99**

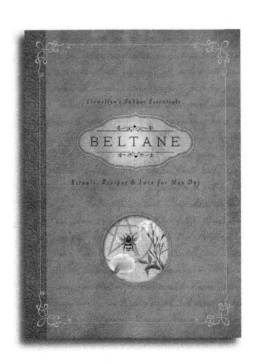

Beltane
Rituals, Recipes & Lore for May Day
LLEWELLYN AND MELANIE MARQUIS

Llewellyn's Sabbat Essentials series explores the old and new ways of celebrating the seasonal rites that are the cornerstones in the witch's year.

A well-rounded introduction to Beltane, this attractive book features rituals, recipes, lore, and correspondences. It includes hands-on information for modern celebrations, spells and divination, recipes and crafts, invocations and prayers, and more!

In agricultural societies, Beltane marked the start of the summer season. We all have something we want to harvest by the end of the year—plans we are determined to realize. Beltane is the time to put our plans into action, and this book will show you how.

978-0-7387-4193-2, 240 pp., 5 x 7   **$11.99**

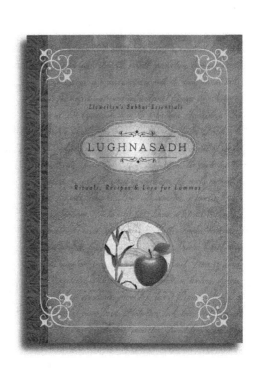

Llewellyn's Sabbat Essentials

LUGHNASADH

Rituals, Recipes & Lore for Lammas

Lughnasadh
Rituals, Recipes & Lore for Lammas
LLEWELLYN AND MELANIE MARQUIS

Lughnasadh—also known as Lammas—is the beginning of the harvest season, marking the point where the first fruit of the land has ripened. This guide to Lughnasadh shows you how to perform rituals and work magic around the gratitude we feel for plans that have come to fruition and explore themes of fertility, protection, and reflection.

Rituals

Recipes

Lore

Spells

Divination

Crafts

Correspondences

Invocations

Prayers

Meditations

978-0-7387-4178-9, 240 pp., 5 x 7   **$11.99**

TENDING BRIGID'S FLAME

AWAKEN TO THE CELTIC GODDESS
OF HEARTH, TEMPLE, AND FORGE

LUNAEA WEATHERSTONE

Tending Brigid's Flame
Awaken to the Celtic Goddess of Hearth, Temple, and Forge
LUNAEA WEATHERSTONE

Brigid is worshiped worldwide as a source of inspiration, protection, and blessing. *In Tending Brigid's Flame*, Lunaea Weatherstone presents the beloved Celtic goddess as a true soul-friend for women today, exploring her legends and lore, attributes and allies, holidays, symbols, and sacred places. Filled with rituals, exercises, and meditations, *Tending Brigid's Flame* shows how to welcome Brigid into your home and make sacred all the activities of everyday life, from food magic to faery traditions, and from scrying to personal healing. Using the symbolism of fires that burn in hearth, temple, and forge, this breathtaking book sends you on a journey through the transformative power of one of the world's most revered goddesses.

978-0-7387-4089-8, 288 pp., 6 x 9 $17.99

HOLISTIC ENERGY MAGIC

———— ✦ ————

Charms & Techniques for Creating a Magical Life

TESS WHITEHURST

Holistic Energy Magic
Charms & Techniques for Creating a Magical Life
TESS WHITEHURST

Perform feats of magic that will energize and activate the desires of your heart. Join Tess Whitehurst as she shows you how to make personal challenges feel less like the end of the world and more like opportunities for magic and new understanding.

Holistic Energy Magic provides important insights into "no tools magic" and the foundations of personal power: intention, visualization, symbolic action, grateful expectation, and alignment with All That Is. Exploring a variety of magical principles and accessible techniques, Tess shows you how to:

Cultivate a relationship with the five elements

Develop your invisible magical toolbox

Create an energetic palette of color, light, crystals, flowers, and sounds

Develop relationships with angels, ancestors, animals, and other allies

Interpret symbols and dreams for a deeper alignment with All That Is

Complete with a spellbook of charms and invocations for protection, serenity, love, and prosperity, this book shares the secrets of attuning your life to the frequency of your truest and most authentic desires.

978-0-7387-4537-4, 288 pp., 5³⁄₁₆ x 8   **$16.99**

To order, call 1-877-NEW-WRLD
Prices subject to change without notice
Order at Llewellyn.com 24 hours a day, 7 days a week!